Praise for **The Complete Family** (

"What a fantastic guide! The book empowers [...]
will get needed answers and guidance, and wa[...]
ies. Relatable, authentic, practical—this is the book I wish I'd had when my
mother was diagnosed."
> —Karen F., Marblehead, Massachusetts

"Two dedicated experts walk caregivers through everything from understanding a loved one's diagnosis to dealing with the entire range of expected
medical, psychiatric, and behavioral issues. Most important, this book is a
guide to building the best possible relationship with the person who is living and even thriving in spite of their cognitive changes."
> —Marc E. Agronin, MD, author of *The End of Old Age:*
> *Living a Longer, More Purposeful Life*

"This book is a lifesaver. In down-to-earth language, it deftly captures the
latest expert advice about dementia care. Dr. Forester brilliantly cared for
my wife with dementia—and taught me, her chief care partner, how to
survive and thrive."
> —Jerry M., Cambridge, Massachusetts

"This wonderful book speaks directly to adult children caring for a parent with dementia, and gives equal weight to the facts, the feelings, and
the often bumpy road to understanding, acceptance, and effective care.
The sections on how to communicate and resolve conflicts with the 'other'
parent—the one who doesn't have dementia—are unique. Above all, this
book shows us how to focus on the feelings—our own, our siblings', and
our parents'—that are at the heart of caregiving but can give us the biggest
challenges."
> —Soo Borson, MD, Professor of Clinical Family
> Medicine, University of Southern California Keck
> School of Medicine; Professor Emerita of Psychiatry
> and Behavioral Sciences, University of Washington

"For the adult child of a parent with dementia, the emotional impact is
unlike any other disease. This reassuring book helps you navigate your new
role in your relationship with your parent and provides concrete, useful
advice for managing common concerns. The authors show how 'working
smarter' can enhance your loved one's quality of life. It is sure to be a
trusted guidebook and companion."
> —Susan W. Lehmann, MD, Clinical Director,
> Division of Geriatric Psychiatry and Neuropsychiatry,
> The Johns Hopkins University School of Medicine

THE COMPLETE FAMILY GUIDE TO DEMENTIA

Also Available

The Complete Family Guide to Addiction:
Everything You Need to Know Now
to Help Your Loved One and Yourself

Thomas F. Harrison and Hilary S. Connery

The
Complete
Family Guide
to Dementia

EVERYTHING YOU NEED
TO KNOW TO HELP YOUR PARENT
AND YOURSELF

Thomas F. Harrison

Brent P. Forester, MD

THE GUILFORD PRESS

New York   London

Copyright © 2022 The Guilford Press
A Division of Guilford Publications, Inc.
370 Seventh Avenue, Suite 1200, New York, NY 10001
www.guilford.com

The information in this volume is not intended as a substitute for consultation with healthcare professionals. Each individual's health concerns should be evaluated by a qualified professional.

Printed in the United States of America

This book is printed on acid-free paper.

Last digit is print number: 9   8   7   6   5   4   3   2   1

Library of Congress Cataloging-in-Publication Data is available from the publisher.

ISBN 978-1-4625-4942-9 (paperback) — ISBN 978-1-4625-4971-9 (hardcover)

Contents

III. Caring Smarter, Not Harder

IV. The Later Stages

Introduction

"My parent has dementia. It's a brain disorder . . . and it's making *me* crazy."

Millions of people can identify with that statement, although they might feel guilty saying it out loud. As life expectancies have rapidly increased, the number of people who live long enough to experience Alzheimer's disease and other forms of dementia has grown enormously. More and more adult children find themselves having to deal with parents who are losing their memories and their ability to function in the world.

Dementia is unique, and caring for someone with dementia is unique too. Coping with a parent with dementia is utterly unlike taking care of someone with a "normal" disease. Children don't just have to deal with the fact that their parents can no longer do many things for themselves; they also have to be on alert every day and night for novel and unexpected ways that their parents might cause problems or get into trouble. The disease is unpredictable—as it progresses, you never know exactly what's going to happen next, and difficult issues always seem to arise at the most inconvenient possible time. Parents with dementia are frequently unwilling or unable to cooperate with the care that their children provide—or even to understand or be grateful for it. In fact they often respond with resistance, suspicion, or hostility. And children often lack emotional support, because no one who hasn't gone through it can truly understand the experience.

The result is that thousands upon thousands of adults in the prime of their lives are stressed beyond belief. And it's hard for them to talk about it, because our society doesn't have a name for what they're going through. But here's a brief list of some very common reactions. If you

1

have a parent with dementia, you'll almost certainly identify with a lot of them:

- They're *anxious* about whether their parent is safe and how they will take care of him or her.

- They're *on constant alert* because they know that their parent could do something dangerous at any time.

- They're *frustrated* that their parent can't do simple tasks and won't cooperate with efforts to help.

- They *spend a lot of time* taking care of their parent at the expense of their own needs.

- They *spend a lot of money* taking care of their parent, or worry that they will have to do so in the future.

- They're occasionally *angry* at their parent for resisting their help or treating them with suspicion and resentment.

- They *feel guilty* about being angry or about not being able to take care of their parent as well as they'd like.

- They *feel helpless* because it's often impossible to figure out how to handle difficult situations.

- They're *embarrassed* because their parent sometimes does things that are socially inappropriate.

- They're *annoyed* with siblings or other relatives who won't help or who offer bad advice.

- They're *depressed* about the toll that the situation has taken on their own life.

- They're *hopeless* because the disease keeps getting worse and seems to have no end.

- If their other parent or stepparent is acting as a primary care provider, they're *worried* about whether the person can handle all the demands.

- They're *lonely* because no one understands what they're going through and they have less and less time for friends.

- Their *work suffers*, or they have to take time off from work.

- They're *afraid* of what will happen as the disease progresses.

- They *feel grief* about losing their relationship with their parent—but they can't process the grief in the way that other people do after a death because their parent is still alive.

This cluster of experiences is very common. There's no name for it, and as a society we don't take it seriously. But we need to begin addressing it.

Why This Book Is Different

There are a number of other books on dementia. Some of them are medical texts. Some are family memoirs. A number of books offer advice on caring for someone with the disease.

The books that offer advice are typically written by expert doctors whose goal is to explain how to provide the best possible care for the patient. Often they contain hundreds and hundreds of excruciatingly detailed instructions designed to create the ideal response to every minor outburst and prevent every conceivable type of harm. These books can be very helpful, but they also have an unfortunate tendency to make caring for a parent with dementia more difficult—because they create the illusion that there's a right way to handle every situation and that it's possible to provide perfect care to a dementia sufferer.

The reality is very different. Often there's no best way to handle a situation. There might not even be a good way—or if there is, there's no way to know it in advance. All you can do is do your best and hope to learn from the experience.

It's also impossible to provide perfect care for a dementia patient. Even a round-the-clock team of highly experienced medical professionals would be unable to deal perfectly with someone with dementia, because the disease itself prevents patients from being able to understand or express their needs—and if patients can't express their needs, it's very difficult to know how to respond. Care providers can't be expected to be mind readers . . . especially when the mind they're trying to read can't clearly formulate the thoughts it wants to communicate.

This book is different from many others because it focuses on *you*—the person trying to deal with a parent with dementia. It's not just another patient-care manual. It's designed to help *you* cope with the situation you're in, with the best possible result for both you and your parent.

Let's face it: People who are looking after a parent with dementia are often exhausted and debilitated, physically, mentally, and emotionally. And those who are exhausted and debilitated are not only going to suffer themselves, but are also going to be unable to provide the best care to a family member with a serious illness. The goal of this book is to help you reconceptualize your role as a care provider so that you can lessen the stress, be healthier and happier, and in the long run provide *better* care for your parent.

Caring Smarter

Of course looking after a parent with dementia will always be a significant burden. But it doesn't always have to be a crushing burden. You may have heard the expression *Work smarter, not harder.* The goal of this book is to help you "care smarter, not harder." It's about finding ways to improve the quality of your parent's life while simultaneously improving the quality of your own.

Is that possible? Yes. But it doesn't happen by chance. It requires a *strategy*.

Consider the following situations:

For Jane, taking care of her elderly mother, Rose, was a series of ever-increasing chores, burdens, and worries. She was so busy taking care of Rose's physical needs that she became highly frustrated when Rose mixed up her medications, refused to eat, or made a scene in public. There were angry confrontations when Rose refused to stop driving. Jane spent untold hours trying to untangle bank accounts and unpaid bills and didn't want to think about what would happen if she couldn't care for Rose at home. It seemed like there was always a crisis, such as when Rose fell and ended up in a rehab facility. Jane struggled just to get through the day; she felt flustered and as though she were going to have a nervous breakdown because her stresses and responsibilities were so overwhelming.

When Sarah's father, Ben, became forgetful, Sarah learned about Alzheimer's disease and what to expect. She took steps as soon as possible to manage his finances and found ways to enlist other people's help for him. She approached caregiving as a set of skills to be learned and developed techniques for communicating with him effectively and responding to his difficult behaviors. She researched care facilities ahead of time. She acknowledged that her relationship with Ben was changing, and she decided that her chief goal was for them to be emotionally close in his waning years. She remembers with happiness that, in the months before he died, she spent a lot of quality time with him holding hands, smiling, and reminiscing.

Simply put, the goal of this book is to help you approach caring for your parent more like Sarah. It's to give you an overall strategy and a series of skills to help you "care smarter." Doing so will not only keep you healthy and preserve your sanity; it will also enable you to provide better, more effective care—and it will lead to a more satisfying and rewarding relationship with your parent in the face of a very challenging illness.

The book starts off with a brief discussion of what dementia is and how it affects the brain. You don't have to be a medical expert to be a good care provider, but understanding the basic nature of the disease will give you a better sense of what you're up against . . . and how and why certain approaches will make life easier down the road.

Part II is about formulating a strategy to deal with the disease. It explains why it's so hard to care for someone with dementia and why people who approach the task without an overall plan so often flounder. It discusses your new relationship with your parent, the different ways in which it's necessary to relate to your parent, and how to set goals for your interactions. It also talks about what can happen if you have another parent or stepparent in the picture.

Part III explains specific skills that you can use to help your parent and make your life easier. You'll learn how to communicate better, how to handle financial and other issues, how to keep your parent safe, and how to get help. You'll also learn how to prevent and deal with problem behaviors (including, occasionally, those of your other family members).

Finally Part IV is about the later stages of the disease, when you can no longer handle everything yourself. You'll learn how to deal with advanced dementia, including how to choose a care facility if necessary and how to make the most of your parent's time there.

No one wants to be in the position of caring for a parent with dementia. But armed with this book, you can approach the task with greater confidence. You can help your parent more effectively, avoid "caregiver burnout," and know in the end that you've had the best relationship you possibly could with your mother or father toward the end of life.

Sadly we can't cure dementia. But with the right approach, we can greatly reduce the stresses caused by having a parent with dementia—and that's a big advantage for everyone.

I

Understanding Your Parent's Dementia

1

What Is Dementia?

How Is It Different from Just Getting Older?

Dementia is a broad name for a group of diseases that cause people to lose their memory and thinking ability. Once people have dementia, it tends to get worse over time; it can eventually become fatal because the brain loses the ability to manage the various bodily functions that keep us alive. In some cases, the process can be slowed down or alleviated, but for right now there is no cure.

What a terrible and uniquely scary problem this is!

There are certainly many other awful illnesses in the world—diabetes, heart disease, kidney failure, and so on—but dementia is different because we don't tend to *identify* with our kidneys or our pancreas. We think of them as a part of our body of course, but we don't consider them to be essential to what makes us who we are. If we received a kidney transplant, we'd still think we were the same person, just with a different kidney. But take away our memory—or, if it were possible, imagine receiving a memory transplant—and we'd feel like we were no longer there at all. Our memory is, in a very large sense, our identity. It's who we are. Dementia doesn't just attack our bodies; it tries to erase our very selves.

And our memory represents our identity for other people too. When people with dementia lose their memory, their family members often remark, "They're no longer the same person they used to be."

Of course a lot of people tend to become more forgetful as they get older, and this forgetfulness can be a normal part of the aging process—the memory function of the brain can slow down in much the same way as other parts of the body do.

But there's a big difference between this "normal" slowing down that often occurs with age and dementia, which is a disease process. In exactly the same way, there's a big difference between naturally becoming less physically active as you get older and developing a disease, such as rheumatism, that damages your muscles or joints.

In the very early stages of dementia though, it can be hard to tell the difference. Dementia can actually start years before it becomes noticeable to other people, even close family members. In fact it can be a very long time before dementia sufferers themselves begin to realize that anything is wrong. Early on, the forgetfulness of dementia may not hinder people's lives very much and can seem like a normal part of getting older.

How You Can Tell

Nevertheless, if you look closer, it's often possible to distinguish between normal aging and early dementia. Dementia affects the brain in a different and characteristic way. The *types* of things that people tend to forget, along with the ways in which they behave regarding them, often provide critical clues.

Perhaps the best way to explain the difference is with a side-by-side comparison. The list below through page 12 should help give you a sense of the difference between occasional age-related forgetfulness and a cognitive problem caused by a disorder in the brain.

Of course this chart is neither exhaustive nor conclusive. Making a few mistakes of the sort described in the right column doesn't amount to proof that someone is a dementia sufferer. However, the comparison is a good way to demonstrate the types of cognitive mistakes that are most typical of dementia.

More likely to be normal aging	*More likely to be dementia*
Not being able to remember a conversation or a decision that took place a year ago.	Not being able to remember a conversation or a decision that took place a day or two ago.
Forgetting the name of a recent or casual acquaintance.	Forgetting the name of an old friend or family member.

More likely to be normal aging	*More likely to be dementia*
Forgetting the date or the day of the week.	Forgetting the year or the month or what season it is. Also being confused about the passage of time.
Occasionally losing things, such as a wallet or car keys.	Losing things in unusual places, such as putting a wallet in the refrigerator or car keys in the medicine cabinet. Also losing things and being unable to retrace one's steps.
Forgetting something and asking someone about it.	Asking the same question over and over.
Forgetting things but being able to remember them with a prompt or clue.	Forgetting things and being unable to remember them even with a prompt or clue.
Occasionally getting confused by a device such as a phone, TV remote, or microwave.	Being unable to remember how to get to a familiar location or the rules of a favorite game.
Sometimes having trouble finding the right word.	Calling things by the wrong name or by a description ("that thing that tells the time") or simply pointing to an object and saying "that thing."
Sometimes forgetting what one was about to say.	Losing the thread of a conversation, suddenly changing the subject, or repeating oneself.
Occasionally forgetting an appointment.	Being highly dependent on written appointment reminders or other memory aids.

More likely to be normal aging	*More likely to be dementia*
Making a mistake in balancing a checkbook.	Using poorer judgment about money in general.
Developing particular ways of doing things and disliking changes in routine.	Larger mood and personality changes, including becoming depressed, suspicious, anxious, or easily upset.
Misty or foggy vision.	Having trouble judging distances or misinterpreting patterns on a carpet or reflections in a mirror.
Making mistakes and being conscious of them.	Making mistakes and not realizing it.

While this list may be helpful, it doesn't substitute for a doctor's diagnosis of dementia. As you'll see in the following chapter, it can be very useful to get a medical diagnosis—particularly because a significant number of cases that *appear* to be dementia in fact have other causes and can be treated or cured.

A Hidden Disease

Older people and their families are often slow to identify dementia early on because it can seem like normal aging, but there are two other reasons dementia frequently goes unrecognized for a long time. (As you'll soon see, these two reasons are also a big part of what makes taking care of a parent with dementia so extraordinarily difficult.)

The first reason is that *the nature of the disease process itself* often causes dementia sufferers to be unaware of the cognitive deficits they're developing. They literally lose the ability to know what they don't know and to remember that they're not remembering things.

The second factor is that dementia sufferers are often in *denial*. Denial is a psychological defense mechanism in which the brain deals with a terrible event or piece of news that would otherwise cause trauma by simply not recognizing or processing it. And of course the idea that you're developing dementia—that you're literally losing your mind—is about as traumatic an idea as one could experience.

A certain amount of denial can be healthy. Denial exists to protect us from experiences that would otherwise be a terrible shock to our psychological and emotional well-being and to allow us to come to terms with traumatic situations in a gradual way, rather than in a sudden and debilitating way.

With dementia, however, a very common result is that people who might otherwise perceive that they're developing memory problems simply begin lying to themselves about it. And they lie to others too or at least unintentionally mislead them, which is a necessary step in remaining in denial.

The way this plays out is that many people in the early stages of dementia engage in elaborate compensations—a kind of "cover-up." They laugh off memory lapses as harmless "senior moments" or instances of just getting older. They may retire from their jobs, not because they're otherwise ready to retire but because they're finding them too difficult. They may gradually let others take on responsibilities, such as paying bills or reconciling bank statements, by saying that they find them unpleasant. They may isolate themselves and avoid new situations that they would experience as challenging. They may claim to no longer like foods that are in fact just complicated to prepare. They may fall back on stock phrases in conversations or consistently turn the topic toward long-term memories or other subjects that they find easier to discuss.

Although family members may develop suspicions, this sort of cover-up can often be successful for an extended period of time. Many people in the early stages of dementia retain a lot of social graces, for instance, and can effectively engage in casual interactions that don't require deep thought or dealing with anything complicated or unusual.

The slow-developing nature of the disease also makes the cover-up harder to spot, especially for spouses who live with the person every day and thus are less apt to notice gradual changes than an adult child who doesn't see the person as frequently.

It's also the case that family members can be in denial themselves. This tends to be especially true of spouses, who often have a very hard time admitting that the person they have loved and lived with for many years is in a process of cognitive decline.

Frequently the way that family members finally realize what's going on is that there's an unusual event or a crisis that puts the person in a situation that can't be handled through the familiar adaptations. The death of a spouse is an extreme example, but the triggering event could be far less dramatic—a family vacation, or the other spouse developing an illness, or some other circumstance in which the person is suddenly forced to handle unexpected responsibilities. All of a sudden it becomes clear that what had previously been passing for normal aging is in fact a brain disease.

Of course waiting for a crisis is never ideal. The sooner you can recognize the disease and begin to plan for it, the better off everyone will be. The next chapter provides some further guidance on how to tell if the changes you're noticing are in fact dementia or have some other cause.

2

How Can I Know for Sure
If My Parent Has Dementia?

It can be a very good idea to have a doctor determine whether your parent has dementia, for a variety of reasons:

- First and most important, in a significant number of cases what looks like dementia actually has another cause—and it might be cured.

- Getting a diagnosis can allow you to begin treatments and practices that may slow the progress of the disease. Many treatments work better the sooner in the disease process the person starts using them.

- Knowing for sure makes it easier for you and your parent to plan for life changes that you'll need to make.

- If your parent is still working, it might make it possible to qualify for disability benefits.

- Having a diagnosis in your parent's medical chart will alert other doctors that they have to be careful with treatment—they can't simply assume that your parent will follow cursory verbal instructions, for instance.

- Having a diagnosis in your parent's chart will also alert doctors not to prescribe certain types of medicines that can have an adverse effect on people with dementia.

Of course it's not always easy to persuade a parent to get tested—and sometimes it's difficult to get other relatives on board as well. This problem is discussed later in this chapter.

How Testing Works

General practitioners or primary care physicians can sometimes diagnose dementia, and they can be a good place to start because they can often administer a simple memory test and check for other medical problems that could be causing memory loss. However, a diagnosis is frequently left up to a specialist, such as a geriatrician, geriatric psychiatrist, or neurologist. You may be able to get a referral from your doctor, a local hospital, or an organization such as the Alzheimer's Association. There are also a growing number of memory clinics that provide a comprehensive clinical assessment, often with a team of doctors to help establish a diagnosis and recommend a treatment plan.

Unfortunately there's no one test or procedure that can give you a definitive yes-or-no answer as to whether someone has dementia. As a result, a diagnosis is usually made through a two-step process: (1) establishing that the person is exhibiting problems and behaviors that are typical of dementia (such as those in the chart in the previous chapter) and (2) ruling out other possible causes for these problems and behaviors.

STEP ONE

Step One involves determining that at least two of the person's core mental functions are impaired enough to interfere with daily living. Core mental functions include the ability to remember things, use language, focus and pay attention, use reason to solve problems, and have accurate visual perception.

As part of Step One, it's often helpful for the doctor to interview family members. People with dementia might be unable to remember or fully articulate the problems they're having, and they might also be in denial.

It's common for doctors to give the person a brief cognitive test, usually lasting 10 minutes or less. There are a number of such tests, but among the most common are the Mini-Mental State Examination (MMSE) and the Montreal Cognitive Assessment (MoCA). Typical tasks include identifying the date and where the person is, recalling words after a delay, repeating complex sentences, drawing a clock face, identifying drawings of animals, copying a geometric figure, and performing simple math.

These two tests result in scores from 0 to 30; the lower the score, the higher the likelihood of dementia.

An even simpler test, called the Mini-Cog, consists of only two tasks: recalling words and drawing a clock face. Despite its simplicity, it has shown fairly good results in diagnosing cognitive impairment. However, compared to the MMSE and MoCA, it's less useful in tracking a person's impairment over time. It's generally easier to judge the degree to which a dementia sufferer is declining by comparing repeated MMSE or MoCA scores.

Another very simple test, called the General Practitioner Assessment of Cognition or GPCOG, is often used by doctors in the United States to flag possible dementia during Medicare patients' annual wellness visits.

While these tests are useful, they're not perfect. For instance, people who aren't native speakers or have a lower educational level may score worse, regardless of their true level of cognition. Also how the test is administered can make a huge difference. Some doctors are very strict, while others tend to give people extra time or hints if they are close, and some are more lenient than others in deciding what is a correct geometric figure or a normal clock face. Also as digital clocks have replaced analog clocks, many people are increasingly unfamiliar with a traditional clock face, and motor difficulties can make it hard to draw a clock or a geometric figure even if the person is cognitively intact. These issues can result in significant scoring fluctuations. Nevertheless the tests are very effective overall in revealing whether someone has a cognitive decline.

More detailed tests, called neuropsychological tests, can delve into specific types of cognitive impairments and may be useful in determining what type of dementia a person has.

STEP TWO

Step Two is by far the more valuable process for family members. After all, by the time parents are brought in for testing, it's usually pretty clear that they're having memory problems. The real question is whether the doctor can find some other, hopefully curable cause of the difficulties.

A thorough Step Two examination will usually involve the following elements. (In the United States, these costs are typically covered by Medicare if the person is 65 or older.)

A Physical Exam and Review of the Person's Medical History. A physical exam and medical history may reveal a number of other diseases that could be causing memory difficulties. For example, heart disease can sometimes interfere with cognitive functioning because of a lack of proper blood flow to the brain. Similarly, chronic obstructive pulmonary disease can cause memory problems because the brain isn't getting enough oxygen from the lungs, and diabetes has also been linked to cognitive impairment.

A medical history can reveal whether any medicines the person is taking might be causing confusion. Some very common and even over-the-counter medications can have this effect, including Benadryl and many pain pills and sleep aids.

Sometimes the problem isn't just a side effect of one medication, but rather a combination of medicines or a combination of medicines and over-the-counter nutritional supplements.

Vision and hearing tests can reveal whether people are having trouble understanding what's going on around them as a result of a loss in vision or hearing.

Another common question is whether there's a family history of dementia, since dementia has a genetic component and a family history makes it more likely.

The doctor may also ask questions about excessive alcohol or drug use. While you might think that problems with alcohol or drugs are unlikely for senior citizens, U.S. government figures show that misuse of alcohol and prescription drugs by the elderly is one of the fastest-growing health problems in the country and affects as many as 17 percent of people over age 60. One study found that among women over 60, binge drinking increased at an average rate of 3.7 percent per year between 1997 and 2014.

Excessive alcohol and drug use can cause problems similar to dementia. Many children would be very reluctant or shocked to think that their parent has such a problem, but it can actually be good news—the brain problems caused by substance abuse are largely reversible, whereas the brain problems caused by dementia are not.

Even if your parent has not increased his or her alcohol intake, people's brains may become more sensitive to alcohol as they age, so that even consuming the same amount of alcohol could result in effects that weren't present before.

You should also note that people who have untreated HIV can develop dementia symptoms, which can often be reversed through medicines called protease inhibitors.

Blood and Urine Testing. This type of testing can reveal a number of other possible causes of memory problems, including poor nutrition, dehydration, anemia, vitamin deficiencies (especially vitamins D, B12, and folate), too much or too little sodium or potassium, thyroid problems, kidney or liver disorders, and a number of degenerative diseases.

A urinary tract infection is another common culprit. These infections can produce symptoms that are very similar to those of dementia, and they can be hard to detect because in older people they often don't result in a fever.

Neurological Testing. Neurological testing includes checking the person's balance, reflexes, eye movements, and so on. These types of tests can reveal signs of a stroke, a brain tumor, Parkinson's disease, hydrocephalus (abnormal accumulation of fluid in the brain), and other illnesses.

Psychological Screening. A psychological screening will look for signs of depression, major stresses or life changes, anxiety disorders, or other problems that can cause symptoms similar to those of dementia.

Brain Scans. Brain scans, most commonly CT scans and MRIs, may reveal evidence of internal bleeding as well as some of the same problems that are checked for with neurological testing.

Another issue is concussions. Many older people are at risk for falls, and if a fall results in a concussion or contusion, it might not be immediately obvious. The person might get up and say that nothing is wrong, but over time the brain injury could lead to significant memory and cognitive issues.

After all these tests have been administered, if there doesn't appear to be any other medical cause for a person's dementia-like symptoms, then the doctor will likely diagnose the person with dementia. Since there's no conclusive test, dementia is usually written up as a "probable" diagnosis, but the probability is actually very high.

Some doctors will try to diagnose a specific type of dementia (as discussed in the next chapter). But others will simply say that the person has dementia generally, often because figuring out the likely specific type would require much more detailed testing.

Not Everyone Wants a Diagnosis

It's not at all uncommon for parents to refuse dementia testing—or even to act insulted at the very suggestion. Part of their refusal may be due to the factors mentioned in the last chapter: The disease itself may make them unaware of their mental lapses, and they may also be in denial.

But there are also rational reasons for resisting testing. Many parents are simply afraid of the consequences. One survey asked seniors why they didn't want to be tested and found that the top reasons were fear of losing their driver's license and fear of upsetting family members. Other significant fears included losing their job, losing their home, losing their long-term care insurance, becoming depressed, and being put in a nursing home.

An additional factor is that there is no cure for dementia. Thus, many seniors may feel that knowing they have the disease offers no real benefit to them that would offset the negative consequences. And of course some seniors would simply be embarrassed by a diagnosis or afraid of the effects of the social stigma that still surrounds the disease.

Several studies of primary care patients who were offered routine dementia screening found that the refusal rates ranged from 7 to 23 percent. However, it's entirely reasonable to assume that the refusal rates among people who *suspected* that they might have dementia were much higher, since these are the very people who would be most motivated to refuse testing because they were afraid of the consequences. And one survey of residents in affluent retirement communities found that only 49 percent would be willing to be regularly screened for dementia.

Another problem is that family members are sometimes opposed to dementia screening. You might think that testing your parent is a good idea, but you might face opposition from your other parent, stepparent, or siblings. These relatives might be in denial themselves, or they might have the same fears we've just described—that a diagnosis will result in financial problems with no clear benefit.

A final irony is that seniors sometimes resist getting a dementia diagnosis primarily because they're afraid that it will upset their family, while families sometimes resist getting a diagnosis because they're afraid that it will upset the senior. Nothing gets done because both sides are scared—often mistakenly—of how a diagnosis will affect the other.

The reality is that, if anything, a dementia diagnosis is often more upsetting to family members than it is to the seniors who have dementia. Seniors with dementia often already have a good idea deep down of what's happening—and in some cases, the disease may have progressed to the point where they don't fully grasp the implications of the diagnosis.

One scientific study found that, contrary to many people's fears, receiving a dementia diagnosis was highly unlikely to cause seniors to become upset or depressed, and in fact both seniors and their family members tended to experience a lot less anxiety once they had a clear explanation for the symptoms along with a treatment plan.

Nevertheless while there are no precise statistics, in actual practice it seems likely that only about half of all dementia cases are ever formally diagnosed, and of the ones that are, the great majority are not diagnosed until the person has moved beyond the early stages and is having marked difficulty with ordinary life activities, such as driving and paying bills.

What You Can Do

If you're having trouble persuading a parent to get a dementia screening, one option is to talk to your parent's doctor and explain the symptoms you're noticing and your parent's (or family's) opposition to testing. The doctor might be willing to skip the cognitive tests in Step One on pages 16–17, relying on your descriptions and a brief conversation with your parent, and proceed with Step Two—ruling out other causes. The doctor's office might simply call to arrange a routine physical exam, and the doctor can then order some follow-up tests, such as blood work and a CT scan or MRI—all without ever specifically mentioning dementia.

In this scenario, you might not get a formal dementia diagnosis, but at least you're accomplishing the most important task of determining whether there's some other medical cause that can be addressed. And if there isn't, at least you'll know to a high degree of certainty that you're dealing with dementia, even if there's no formal statement in the charts.

One more tip: If you *are* able to get a formal dementia diagnosis from a doctor, it's important to include your parent fully in the discussion that follows. Dementia sufferers are prone to paranoia, and if parents feel that their children are talking about them in the third person or having a secret conversation with the doctor, it can trigger a very negative reaction. You might well have questions for the doctor that you don't want to discuss in front of your parent, but a better approach is to let the doctor know about your concerns in advance and then follow up privately later.

3

What Causes Memory Loss?

Alzheimer's Disease and the Many Other Causes

Many people think of Alzheimer's disease and dementia as the same thing, but they're not. Alzheimer's disease is one particular type of dementia, but there are a number of others. However, Alzheimer's disease is by far the most common type and accounts for most of the cases.

If it's possible to have a doctor determine which type of dementia your parent has, it can be very useful, because different types can have somewhat different symptoms and can progress differently. Also, some medications that work well for one type might not be recommended for another type.

Treatment can be complicated, however, because many people have more than one problem. In fact, in 2018 a group of scientists conducted autopsies of more than 1,000 people who had suffered from dementia and found that an enormous number—78 percent—had evidence of two or more dementia types, at least to some extent. And while Alzheimer's was the most common disease and was present in 65 percent of the subjects, only 9 percent of the subjects suffered *only* from Alzheimer's.

Here's a brief look at the different diseases that can result in the symptoms of dementia.

Mild Cognitive Impairment

Mild cognitive impairment, or MCI, is like a "mini" version of dementia. It generally has the same causes as other types of dementia, and it produces the same symptoms, except that the symptoms are not as severe.

The key difference is that, with MCI, memory loss might be frustrating, but it doesn't rise to the level of significantly interfering with a person's activities of daily life. (Remember that in order to diagnose dementia, a doctor has to find that the person's core mental functions are impaired enough to interfere with daily living.)

A lot of people who develop MCI go on to develop dementia. According to the Mayo Clinic, each year about 10 to 15 percent of people with MCI develop full-blown dementia (compared to only about 1 to 3 percent of older adults who don't have MCI). However, MCI doesn't always result in dementia; many people with MCI never develop it, and in some cases the MCI simply "clears up" and the person goes back to normal.

Another feature of MCI is that, compared to dementia, it usually involves a more limited set of symptoms.

Broadly speaking, there are two types of MCI: *amnestic* and *nonamnestic*. People with amnestic MCI suffer from memory loss. They may forget words or appointments or lose things or their train of thought more often than other people their age. However, they won't necessarily have difficulty with other cognitive processes, such as those involved in reconciling a bank statement.

People with nonamnestic MCI are the reverse. They might not have much trouble with memory, but they will experience increased difficulty with planning, decision making, following instructions, finding their way around, and using good judgment.

It's possible though for a person to have both types of MCI at the same time.

(By the way, the "bible" of psychiatric diagnosis in the United States is the American Psychological Association's *Diagnostic and Statistical Manual of Mental Disorders.* In the most recent edition of the manual— the fifth—MCI was renamed *mild neurocognitive disorder.* Dementia itself was renamed *major neurocognitive disorder.* But most people continue to use the terms MCI and *dementia,* and this book will as well.)

Alzheimer's Disease

Alzheimer's disease is the most common cause of dementia, and it's been estimated that it's responsible for as many as two-thirds or even three-quarters of all dementia cases—although it's impossible to come up with a precise figure. It's believed that there are currently about 6 million cases of Alzheimer's in the United States, and the number is expected to reach 15 million by 2050.

Unlike MCI, Alzheimer's affects all areas of cognition, including memory, judgment, planning, orientation, visual perception, and motor skills. However, memory problems are usually the first sign that people notice.

The disease is progressive, meaning that it gets worse over time. It's ultimately fatal, although the course of the disease varies tremendously from person to person; it can lead to death in as little as 3 years or as many as 20 or more—and determining this length of time is itself very difficult, because the disease begins so gradually and its early symptoms are so similar to normal aging that it's often very difficult to determine exactly when it started.

In any event, because Alzheimer's is a lengthy disease and it primarily strikes people who are old to begin with, it's not uncommon for them to die of some other natural cause first.

Alzheimer's disease works by killing nerve cells in the brain. A healthy brain contains billions of nerve cells, or neurons, that communicate, organize, and store information. In a person with Alzheimer's, these cells are attacked by two culprits, known as plaques and tangles:

- Neuritic plaques are deposits of a protein called beta-amyloid in the spaces between neurons.

- Neurofibrillary tangles are twisted fibers of a protein called tau inside of neurons.

Occasional plaques and tangles develop fairly commonly in older people, which is one reason that people's memory naturally slows down with aging. However, in the brains of people with Alzheimer's disease, the plaques and tangles build up systematically, and they aggressively attack the neurons, usually starting with the ones devoted to memory and spreading to other areas of the brain.

While we have a fairly good idea of how Alzheimer's disease works, there are a couple things we don't know. One is how to determine *for sure* if a person has the disease. There is no test that can definitively show if a person has the plaques-and-tangles pattern characteristic of Alzheimer's. In fact, the only way to be 100 percent sure is through an autopsy. (This is one reason we can't determine the exact percentage of dementia cases for which Alzheimer's is responsible.)

Nevertheless doctors who diagnose "probable" Alzheimer's tend to be correct the vast majority of the time. A very likely diagnosis can be made on the basis of characteristic symptoms, the progression of the symptoms over time, and ruling out other possible causes.

We also don't know what causes the buildup of plaques and tangles in the first place. Genetics plays a role, and certain genes have been identified as increasing the likelihood of getting Alzheimer's. Consistent with this observation, studies have shown that people with a family history of Alzheimer's are more likely to develop it themselves. However, plenty of people who have the "suspect" genes never get Alzheimer's, and plenty of people who don't have the suspect genes do get it, so other factors are clearly at work too.

An interesting question is why the disease typically strikes people over 65. Some theories suggest that the disease results from an interaction between genetic susceptibility and natural changes that occur in the brain as people get older. (There's evidence that amyloid plaques can begin accumulating in the brain 15 to 20 years before a person has enough symptoms to be diagnosed.)

However, about 5 percent of Alzheimer's cases arise when people are significantly younger, so there appear to be other causes and genetic complexities as well.

It has also been shown that Alzheimer's disease is more common in people who smoke, are exposed to air pollution, or have certain gum diseases.

The disease is named for Alois Alzheimer, a German doctor who extensively studied the case of a patient named Auguste Deter. When Deter died in 1906, Alzheimer performed an autopsy and discovered the presence of the telltale plaques and tangles.

Lewy Body Dementia

Lewy bodies are abnormal protein aggregates that can develop inside neurons. They're different from the plaques and tangles of Alzheimer's.

Lewy bodies can appear in the parts of the brain that govern motor functions, and they can also appear in the parts that govern cognitive functions. Sometimes they will spread from the motor areas to the cognitive areas.

When Lewy bodies attack the motor parts of the brain, the result is called Parkinson's disease. When they attack the cognitive parts, leading to dementia, the result is called *dementia with Lewy bodies.* If Lewy bodies spread from the motor areas to the cognitive areas, the condition is called *Parkinson's disease with dementia.*

The general term *Lewy body dementia* includes both dementia with Lewy bodies and Parkinson's disease with dementia.

As with Alzheimer's disease, there is no definitive test for Lewy body dementia—the only way to know for sure is an autopsy. However, it can be important to try to distinguish the two, because the types of antipsychotic medications that are sometimes given to Alzheimer's sufferers who experience delusions or hallucinations can cause very adverse reactions in people with Lewy body dementia.

Key differences between Alzheimer's disease and Lewy body dementia include the following:

- People with Lewy body dementia are far more likely to experience visual hallucinations, and they typically occur much earlier in the disease process than is common with Alzheimer's.

- People with Lewy body dementia often have *fluctuating cognition*, meaning that they may have a very high level of alertness for several days and then have a very different level of alertness for several days. This condition is much less common in Alzheimer's.

- People with Lewy body dementia often have Parkinson's-like symptoms, including stiffness, slow movements, tremors, muscle weakness, stooped posture, a shuffling gait, a blank facial expression, small handwriting, and a general lack of balance and dexterity. (Alzheimer's sufferers also typically develop a lack of balance, but not until later in the disease process.)

People with Lewy body dementia may experience elaborate and systematized delusions. They may also suffer from sleep problems, including interrupted sleep due to vivid dreams, "acting out" while dreaming, restless legs syndrome, and excessive daytime sleeping.

Although the early symptoms of Lewy body dementia can be significantly different from those of Alzheimer's disease, the symptoms of the two diseases tend to become much more similar as they progress.

Vascular Dementia

Vascular dementia is caused by damage to the brain resulting from a large stroke, a series of smaller strokes, or inflammation of blood vessels. Vascular dementia is different from Alzheimer's disease and Lewy body dementia in that it only affects one specific part of the brain. The symptoms vary and depend on what part of the brain has been damaged, but the most common problems involve memory, coordination, and speech. Depression is also a frequent symptom.

Another key difference from Alzheimer's is that there is often a sudden onset of memory problems, as opposed to a gradual loss. Also while Alzheimer's is a progressive disease, people with vascular dementia don't always get worse over time. And if they *do* get worse, it tends to happen suddenly. The pattern is "plateaus and cliffs," as opposed to a continual decline.

As compared to Alzheimer's sufferers, people with vascular dementia are more likely to experience nighttime confusion, dizziness, and sudden mood changes. They are also likely to retain and express their underlying personality for a longer time.

People who suffer from vascular dementia tend to have difficulty *retrieving* information from their memory, whereas people who suffer from Alzheimer's tend to have difficulty *storing* information in their memory. The way this expresses itself is that people with vascular dementia are much more likely to be able to recall things if they're given cues, prompts, or reminders. That's because their challenge is in bringing things out of their memory—whereas with Alzheimer's sufferers, it's as though the information has simply been wiped from their memory.

LATE

Something that has puzzled scientists for a long time is that a significant number of people have symptoms that appear very similar to those of Alzheimer's, but their brains don't have the telltale plaques and tangles associated with the disease. In 2019 a group of scientists proposed that these people actually have a different disease, called *limbic-predominant age-related TDP-43 encephalopathy*, or LATE for short.

LATE could account for as many as 17 percent of all dementia cases, these scientists speculated.

Instead of plaques and tangles, LATE is caused by a dysfunction in a protein called TDP-43. This dysfunction can result, among other things, in a shrinking of the hippocampus, an important part of the brain for regulating memory.

True to its name, LATE tends to occur in older people, especially those over 80. The scientists believe it's possible that a quarter of all people over 85 have enough TDP-43 problems to interfere with memory and cognition to at least some extent.

There's currently no good way to distinguish Alzheimer's from LATE (except through an autopsy), and in fact there's little practical need for family members to do so. The symptoms are similar and the methods of providing care are no different. Also many current medications for Alzheimer's target symptoms rather than the underlying plaques and tangles, and it appears that they will work just as well for people with LATE.

For scientists though distinguishing the two could become very important as medicines are developed that treat the underlying causes of cognitive loss.

Other Types of Dementia

Here are some other, much less common disorders that can also cause dementia symptoms:

• *Frontotemporal dementia* refers to a group of diseases that cause cell loss and shrinkage in the frontal and temporal lobes of the brain. These diseases tend to progress more rapidly than Alzheimer's and tend to fall into two groups. One group results in aphasia—an inability to use and understand speech. The other causes behavioral problems; otherwise well-adjusted people may lose their "censor" and begin behaving in socially inappropriate ways or may become highly apathetic and withdraw from regular activities.

• *Wernicke–Korsakoff syndrome* is caused by a vitamin B1 deficiency. It's commonly associated with alcoholism, although it can also be triggered by eating disorders and chemotherapy. Frequent symptoms include memory problems, disorientation, and difficulty with vision. However, the disease seldom causes language difficulties.

- *Chronic traumatic encephalopathy* is a disease caused by repeated head injuries that produces symptoms of dementia. It often develops 8 to 10 years after the injuries occur. Most cases that have been studied involve people who played contact sports (such as soccer, rugby, football, boxing, and ice hockey), military personnel, and victims of domestic violence.

- *Progressive supranuclear palsy* is a rare disorder caused by a deterioration of cells in the brain stem. It primarily affects balance and vision, but it can also result in memory and language problems and trouble with judgment and problem solving. It may be related to frontotemporal dementia.

- *Cortico-basal ganglionic degeneration* is another rare disorder that may be related to frontotemporal dementia.

- *Creutzfeldt–Jakob disease* is a rare brain disease that causes memory, vision, balance, and behavioral problems. It mostly affects older adults and often leads to death within a year or two.

- *Huntington's disease* is a rare genetic disorder that causes dementia and motor problems. It usually strikes people between the ages of 30 and 50.

- *HIV/AIDS* can cause dementia, although modern drugs called protease inhibitors usually relieve these symptoms. But dementia can still occur in patients who don't take these drugs or who have a form of the disease that is resistant to them.

- *Alcoholism.* People who have had an alcohol use disorder for an extended period of time sometimes develop symptoms of dementia, although the reasons are not well understood.

Will You Get It Too?

Adult children who are taking care of a parent with dementia often become worried that they will somehow inherit the disease. Because they're highly conscious of memory loss all the time, if they happen to forget someone's name or make another type of routine mistake, they might think, "Oh my God, it's happening to me!"

This concern is natural, but these lapses are usually nothing to worry about. It's true that there's a genetic component to dementia, but the genetic basis is very complicated and is particularly pronounced only with certain forms of the illness such as frontotemporal dementia, Huntington's disease, and "early-onset" Alzheimer's (meaning that the person showed symptoms before the age of 60). If you have a parent or grandparent who developed Alzheimer's disease after age 75, you do not have a markedly increased risk of developing it yourself.

Vascular dementia typically has no genetic component. However, a person who develops vascular dementia as a result of a stroke or other problem could pass down genes that make a child more susceptible to strokes or heart disease.

Large-scale studies have shown that there are a number of risk factors other than genetics that tend to correlate with developing dementia later in life, including diabetes and certain psychiatric problems, such as depression, bipolar disorder, and posttraumatic stress disorder. Other problems that appear to correlate with a greater risk of developing dementia include hypertension, high cholesterol, lack of exercise, heavy alcohol use, and social isolation. The good news is that these are all modifiable risk factors, which means that you can lower your chances of getting dementia simply by living a healthier lifestyle.

4

What to Expect

How the Problem Typically Progresses

A lot of people have tried to think about dementia in terms of stages: They will talk about people having early or mild dementia, moderate dementia, severe or late-stage dementia, and so on.

These terms are a useful shorthand; they can allow you to quickly express how much difficulty the person generally has with daily activities and how much care is needed. However, it's important to remember that dementia is most often a progressive disease that involves a continual, gradual decline. There's no clear dividing line between "mild" and "moderate" dementia, for instance. Some people will have "mild" problems in one cognitive area and "moderate" problems in another. In addition the disease is highly variable: It's entirely possible for someone to have only "mild" difficulties early in the day and to have much more significant problems later in the evening.

Overall though, especially with Alzheimer's disease, it's possible to broadly track a typical progression from when the problem first becomes noticeable to its later stages.

Having a sense of how the disease progresses can be very helpful because it allows you to see what's coming and gives you an opportunity to prepare for it.

And as you'll see in later chapters, *preparation is key*. A great many adult children spend all their time focusing on how to deal with their parent's current symptoms. Then when a new symptom develops, or an existing symptom gets worse, they're surprised and unprepared. They have to begin figuring out how to cope with *that* problem and often, by the time they do, another new problem arises. As a result, they are always behind the curve and struggling to catch up. This is a major reason why taking care of a parent with cognitive decline is so stressful for so many people.

A key theme of this book is learning how to care smarter, not harder—and understanding the course of the disease and what to expect is essential to caring smarter.

The First Signs

The most common first sign of dementia is trouble with memory. The person may have trouble recalling information, finding the right word, keeping appointments, or following the thread of a conversation.

Other early symptoms of dementia include the following:

- Language problems, such as using the wrong word and not real-izing it.

- Losing things, especially misplacing them in inappropriate places.

- Difficulty with complex tasks, such as following a recipe or man-aging finances.

- Being disoriented as to time, such as thinking it's 8:00 A.M. when it's 8:00 P.M.

- Being disoriented as to place, such as having trouble finding a familiar location.

- Trouble focusing or concentrating.

- Poorer judgment than usual.

- Moodiness and personality changes, which can include a general sense of apathy but also anger, swearing, or a lack of inhibition.

Moderate Dementia

A number of symptoms tend to develop later on as the person's condition worsens. They can include having trouble judging distances, distortions of visual perception, delusions or hallucinations, lack of balance and coordination, and loss of the sense of smell.

However, in general, the symptoms of moderate dementia are the same as those of early or mild dementia—except that they become more pronounced and debilitating. The difference is not that the person has different problems; it's that the problems begin interfering more and more with the person's ability to cope with daily living.

Personality changes can become more pronounced too. Some people with dementia become increasingly withdrawn, but it's very common for parents to become anxious, fearful, suspicious, argumentative, petulant, or paranoid. These changes can be very upsetting to children who aren't prepared for them.

The effects of these negative personality changes are often described as *problem behaviors*. They can involve a stubborn refusal to do simple tasks, such as eating or bathing, becoming defensive or arguing for no good reason, blaming you for something that isn't your fault, extreme fear or suspicion, saying or doing something that is highly socially inappropriate, and experiencing hallucinations or delusions. (Dealing with problem behaviors is discussed in Chapters 18–20.)

Problem behaviors aside, what follows is a list of activities that people typically begin losing the ability to handle as their condition gets worse. As you'll see, these are all things that are wise to prepare for ahead of time. If you wait until there's a crisis, and it suddenly becomes obvious that your parent can no longer handle them, you'll be at a significant loss if you haven't thought about what to do in advance.

Working. Many people retire or lose their jobs after they develop dementia, either because they make too many mistakes or because they realize that they will no longer be able to meet the job requirements.

Driving. Driving a car requires multiple skills: motor coordination, quick reflexes, judging speed and distance, following rules, remembering routes, and the ability to coordinate all these skills at the same time. Unfortunately dementia targets every one of these skills. As a result, dementia sufferers often become unsafe behind the wheel—and they may get to this point long before they themselves realize it.

Cooking. Preparing a meal requires conceptualizing and executing a series of logical steps, which is something that people with dementia find very difficult. Some people with dementia begin relying on simple foods that they don't have to cook or foods that they can microwave. Sadly these foods are often unhealthy choices, which can lead to poor nutrition and related health problems. Difficulty with cooking can be dangerous in other ways too—parents might eat a food that has gone bad because of their disorientation about time and diminished sense of smell. Some people will put a pan on the stove and forget about it, which can cause a fire.

Managing Finances. People with dementia typically lose the ability to manage their finances. Not being able to balance a checkbook or otherwise reconcile accounts is an early sign, but as the disease gets worse, they may forget to pay bills, misplace credit cards, lose track of accounts or investments, and make poor financial decisions in general. They are also much more likely to fall for financial scams.

Managing Medications. Confusion, forgetfulness, and disorientation as to time can make it extremely difficult to keep on a medication schedule. A problem with scheduling is dangerous, since a parent may skip important medicines or take them too frequently.

Walking Unassisted. The lack of balance, coordination, and depth perception that accompanies dementia—not to mention confusion, disorientation, and trouble judging distances—can make older people very vulnerable to falling. Parents often need a cane or a walker to get around safely. Unfortunately, of course, the disease can frequently cause them to forget to use it or forget how to use it properly.

Personal Hygiene. At this stage, many people forget or become reluctant to bathe regularly. They may also have difficulty with brushing their teeth, combing their hair, shaving, and dressing appropriately.

Talking on the Phone. Using a telephone can be a significant challenge for dementia sufferers. That's partly because they have trouble recalling phone numbers and remembering how to use the device. In addition a phone call is a much more abstract experience than an in-person conversation—a parent can't rely on body language, facial expressions, and other nonverbal cues to help understand the person's meaning. As a result, troubles with language and following the thread of a conversation are greatly magnified on the phone.

Watching Television. As with phones, dementia sufferers may have trouble operating the equipment, especially as TV remotes become smaller and more complicated. In addition some people who are prone to delusional thinking may get confused and have trouble distinguishing television programs from real life.

Living Alone. Add up all of these problems, and the result is that a parent who is used to living alone may no longer be able to do so safely. This is especially true since people with moderate dementia can be prone to wandering into unfamiliar environments.

Later Stages

In the later stages of dementia, all these problems still exist but in an extreme form. Parents may no longer be able to meaningfully use or understand language, and communication for the most part will be emotional and nonverbal. They may have great difficulty walking and be unable to dress or bathe themselves. They may need a lot of help eating. They may develop problems with incontinence.

Typically they need round-the-clock care. Some adult children heroically try to provide this kind of care, but doing so is a crushing burden and generally proves to be impossible without significant outside help.

Does the Type of Dementia Matter?

This description of the stages of dementia is particularly true of Alzheimer's disease, which is the most common form. As noted in the preceding chapter, with other types of dementia the course of the disease can be somewhat different.

With Lewy body dementia, for instance, you're more likely to have to deal with motor difficulties, hallucinations, and delusions early on in the disease process. And with vascular dementia, you're more likely to experience symptoms suddenly getting worse rather than a pattern of gradual decline.

One scientific study found that families of people with vascular dementia had a much greater caregiving burden in the early stages of the disease compared with families of people with Alzheimer's, but in the later stages the opposite was true.

Nevertheless the burden is serious for any type of dementia. And no matter the type, preparing ahead of time for your parent's future loss of abilities is a key to caring smarter—and to staying sane yourself.

5

Can Dementia Be Treated to Make It Less Severe?

There's no definitive cure for dementia, but there are a number of treatments that may relieve some of the symptoms at least for a while.

A few drugs on the market are designed to slow the decline in cognition and function caused by dementia and have been approved by the U.S. Food and Drug Administration (FDA) for this purpose. Other drugs haven't been specifically approved by the FDA for treating dementia but are sometimes used off-label to address particular behavioral and psychological symptoms of the disease. And there are also psychotherapy approaches that are intended to help dementia sufferers.

This chapter discusses some of the most important options for treatment. You'll want to consult a doctor about these treatments, but having a general overview will help you better understand what's being prescribed and allow you to have a more fruitful interaction with the physician.

Drugs for Dementia

The most common drugs that are used for dementia are called *cholinesterase inhibitors*. These drugs increase the amount of a neurotransmitter in the brain called acetylcholine, which helps brain cells communicate with each other. (People with dementia typically have a reduced amount of acetylcholine.)

As a result of increasing the amount of acetylcholine, dementia sufferers may be better able to remember things and to perform complex tasks. The drugs can also improve behavioral symptoms, reduce hallucinations, and lessen feelings of apathy.

However, these drugs won't revive lost brain cells; they'll simply make the remaining brain cells work more efficiently. Also the drugs won't slow down the progression of the disease. Thus while they might help improve symptoms for a time, after a while they'll cease to provide much benefit because the disease will continue to damage the brain's neurons.

The effect of these drugs is variable. Some people have a marked improvement, but some experience little if any difference.

In the United States, three cholinesterase inhibitors have been approved by the FDA for use with patients with dementia. They are as follows:

Donepezil (Aricept) is a tablet that is taken once per day. It's usually started at a low dose and increased gradually if necessary. Some people take it at bedtime, but taking it in the morning with food can reduce side effects such as gastrointestinal problems, nightmares, and insomnia.

Galantamine (Razadyne) comes in tablet, liquid, and time-release capsule form. The liquid or tablet is taken twice a day; the capsule is taken once a day. Since the drug can cause an upset stomach, it's recommended that it be taken with a meal and that the patient drink plenty of water throughout the day.

Rivastigmine (Exelon) can be taken orally but it sometimes causes nausea, vomiting, and loose stools. The drug is also available as a patch that allows it to be absorbed directly into the bloodstream, which has been shown to reduce these problems.

(A fourth drug called tacrine, or Cognex, was withdrawn from use in the United States in 2013 because it causes a risk of liver injury.)

All these drugs can cause minor side effects, which may include nausea, dizziness, reduced appetite, muscle cramping, tremors, and weight loss. In rare cases the side effects can include a slower heartbeat, gastrointestinal bleeding, and ulcers.

If a patient doesn't improve with one cholinesterase inhibitor, doctors will often switch and try another. However, it's not advisable to use more than one of the drugs at the same time. Since the drugs work in the same general way, using more than one won't increase the effectiveness but might make the side effects worse.

NAMENDA

Another drug called memantine (Namenda) takes a different approach by reducing the effect of a neurotransmitter called glutamate. It's believed that too much glutamate activity in the brain can cause neurons to die or become less able to communicate with each other.

Like cholinesterase inhibitors, Namenda may make it easier for dementia sufferers to remember things and perform complex tasks. However, as with the other drugs, the effects can vary considerably from person to person and the drug won't stop the progression of the disease, which means that after a while it ceases to be effective.

Namenda can be taken either once or twice a day. Common side effects include dizziness, headache, constipation, and confusion.

A newer product called Namzaric combines both Namenda and Aricept.

Another drug, called aducanumab (Aduhelm), was approved by the FDA in 2021. It is discussed later in this chapter.

WHAT TYPES OF DEMENTIA DO THESE DRUGS HELP?

Razadyne and Exelon have been approved to treat mild and moderate Alzheimer's disease, and Aricept has been approved to treat mild, moderate, and severe Alzheimer's.

The effectiveness of cholinesterase inhibitors for types of dementia *other* than Alzheimer's is uncertain. Exelon has been approved by the FDA for use with Parkinson's disease with dementia. And some studies have shown that cholinesterase inhibitors are effective for Lewy body dementia.

The evidence for the use of the drugs with vascular dementia is unclear. Also many people who have vascular dementia are also taking heart medications, and there may be a risk of adverse drug interactions between cholinesterase inhibitors and common heart medicines.

Unfortunately cholinesterase inhibitors don't seem to provide any benefit to people with frontotemporal dementia.

As for Namenda, it has been approved for moderate and severe Alzheimer's disease. The evidence is mixed for milder forms of the disease, although a recent small study suggested that it might help with MCI. Namenda hasn't been approved for Lewy body or vascular dementia, but a number of studies have shown that it can be effective, and some doctors will prescribe it off-label to such patients. Not much research has been conducted on whether Namenda helps with frontotemporal dementia, but so far there is very little evidence that it does.

HOW LONG SHOULD THEY BE TAKEN?

All these drugs can be expensive; in the United States, they can cost hundreds of dollars a month, although insurance may help defray the cost.

When using these drugs, it's important to limit your expectations. Even when they work, the disease will continue to progress, so any positive effect will typically last only a few months or a year. And when the drugs work, that doesn't mean that the patient's cognitive decline will be reversed; it means that the patient's cognitive decline will be stabilized and there will be a period when the problems won't get noticeably worse for a while.

In general starting the drugs as early as possible can be advisable since doing so may help preserve a higher level of cognitive ability.

Since the drugs can be expensive and since they don't work indefinitely, there can be a significant question about when to stop using them. Many doctors are reluctant to proactively discontinue a prescription as long as the patient has some significant mental functioning, especially since there's no definitive way to tell when they cease working—even if the patient is starting to decline despite the drug, it's impossible to say if the decline would have been worse without it. Sometimes a drug is discontinued, and the patient experiences a more rapid deterioration afterward.

However, the drugs can become cost-prohibitive for many people, and it's the case that some families end up paying for an expensive medication long after it has stopped providing any significant benefit.

It should be noted that there are a few doctors who don't like to prescribe these drugs at all. Because the drugs don't make anyone "better" and it's impossible to measure how much good they actually do, these doctors don't believe they produce a meaningful result.

ADUHELM

In 2021 the FDA approved a controversial new drug called aducanumab, or Aduhelm, which its manufacturer Biogen claims is the first medicine capable of attacking Alzheimer's disease itself—by reducing amyloid plaques in the brain—rather than just ameliorating the symptoms of dementia. Aduhelm was approved for mild Alzheimer's dementia and MCI.

The approval of Aduhelm caused a backlash among scientists who felt that there simply wasn't enough clinical evidence that it slowed the cognitive and functional decline associated with Alzheimer's. The decision prompted at least two congressional investigations and caused the FDA's acting commissioner to call for the Justice Department's inspector general's office to look into the approval process. Three members of an FDA review panel resigned after the agency approved the drug despite the panel's recommendation to the contrary.

The American Neurological Association issued a press release saying the drug shouldn't have been approved without additional evidence that it made a difference, although the association supported further clinical trials. On the other hand, the president of the Alzheimer's Association stated that he "welcomes and celebrates the historic FDA approval of aducanumab."

Adding to the controversy was the drug's high cost: Biogen announced that a year's supply of the drug would cost $56,000, although it later lowered the price to $28,200. And Medicare announced that it wouldn't cover the drug unless it was being taken as part of a clinical trial. In addition an initial PET scan or spinal tap would be required, and insurance coverage for this procedure could vary.

OTHER DRUGS

There are some other drugs that are not specifically designed for dementia but are sometimes used to treat dementia-related behavioral and psychological symptoms. They include the following:

Anxiety Drugs. The most common anti-anxiety drugs are benzodiazepines, a category that includes alprazolam (Xanax), lorazepam (Ativan), clonazepam (Klonopin), diazepam (Valium), and temazepam (Restoril). While these drugs may sometimes be helpful in calming down a dementia patient in the moment, they must be used very carefully and should generally be prescribed only for a very limited duration, if at all. They can cause an acute condition called delirium and actually worsen some of the cognitive symptoms of dementia. They can also lead to addiction and an increased risk of falling in the elderly.

Antidepressant Drugs. The most common drugs used to relieve depression are selective serotonin reuptake inhibitors, or SSRIs. These increase the amount of the neurotransmitter serotonin in the brain. Common SSRI medications include citalopram (Celexa), escitalopram (Lexapro), trazodone (Desyrel), sertraline (Zoloft), fluoxetine (Prozac), and paroxetine (Paxil). Other antidepressant drugs include venlafaxine (Effexor), bupropion (Wellbutrin), and mirtazapine (Remeron).

SSRIs can also relieve anxiety and agitation in people with Alzheimer's disease.

Sleep Drugs. Drugs designed to help patients sleep better include zolpidem (Ambien), zaleplon (Sonata), and eszopiclone (Lunesta). Some other drugs are often prescribed off-label for insomnia, including mirtazapine (Remeron), nortriptyline (Pamelor), and gabapentin (Neurontin). Temazepam (Restoril), one of the anxiety drugs, is also prescribed for sleep, and trazodone, one of the antidepressant drugs, is prescribed for sleep under the name Oleptro.

Again these drugs may be helpful, but there are questions about their long-term use, especially in the case of Pamelor, which can block acetylcholine and generally shouldn't be given to patients with dementia.

Melatonin, an over-the-counter sleep aid, has been shown to help reduce sleep irregularity in people with dementia. It may also help with *sundowning* (the tendency of patients with dementia to become increasingly agitated in the evening).

Antipsychotic Drugs. These drugs are sometimes given to patients with dementia who have significant delusions or hallucinations, severe agitation, or behavioral problems. Haloperidol (Haldol) is an older antipsychotic drug that can have very serious side effects. A newer group of what are called atypical antipsychotics includes olanzapine (Zyprexa), quetiapine (Seroquel), clozapine (Clozaril), aripiprazole (Abilify), risperidone (Risperdal), and ziprasidone (Geodon).

Haldol's side effects can include tremors, difficulty walking, and tardive dyskinesia, an involuntary movement disorder. But even the atypical antipsychotic drugs can have significant side effects, including sedation, gait problems, and dizziness when standing up quickly, and they have been associated with an increased risk of stroke and a higher rate of mortality in general. For this reason, if they're used at all, it's usually best to start with a very low dose and try to limit the duration as much as possible. Also antipsychotics might not truly be necessary if the person is experiencing delusions or hallucinations but isn't terribly upset by them.

Antipsychotics are especially a problem with Lewy body dementia, because they can cause serious health risks. Many doctors believe that Seroquel is the least risky antipsychotic for patients with Lewy body dementia. To be safe Seroquel is sometimes given even to patients who have been diagnosed with Alzheimer's disease rather than Lewy body dementia if there's some risk that they *might* have Lewy bodies (since there's no completely definitive test for which type of dementia a person has).

Some cholinesterase inhibitors, especially Exelon, may help reduce visual hallucinations in people with Lewy body dementia.

CBD. CBD, or cannabidiol, is derived from the same plant that produces marijuana but it doesn't get people "high." In the United States, it's legal in virtually every state. Several studies have suggested that the drug can slow the decline of cognitive function in people with dementia and can also calm them down and reduce anxiety, agitation, and behavioral problems. However, the research is very recent, and the FDA hasn't approved any CBD products for use with dementia. CBD is still somewhat controversial, and there is very little oversight of claims being made by some manufacturers about its efficacy and health benefits.

Along the same lines, there are two synthetic cannabinoids that have been approved by the FDA for treating nausea and vomiting associated with cancer chemotherapy: dronabinol (Marinol) and nabilone (Cesamet). There is some evidence that these drugs may also reduce agitation in people with Alzheimer's disease.

Psychotherapy Approaches

Many people are surprised at the idea of psychotherapy for dementia, mainly because the common perception of psychotherapy is an hour in a therapist's office talking about interpersonal problems. The idea of a "talking cure" doesn't make a lot of sense when the patient has a lot of difficulty talking in the first place and is unlikely to remember what was discussed.

With patients who suffer from dementia, the goal of psychotherapy is not to cure them but simply to help them feel calmer, happier, and more oriented to their surroundings. Most such psychotherapy happens in dedicated dementia-care facilities.

The most common approaches include:

Art and activity therapy can improve patients' cognitive functioning and mood. Music seems to work especially well, but other variations include making artworks and crafts, dance, aromatherapy, and pet visits.

Reminiscence therapy tries to improve cognition and mood by encouraging patients to recall positive past experiences, such as family holidays and weddings.

Reality orientation uses signs and other information to remind patients of their immediate surroundings in order to reduce disorientation and confusion. This tends to work best with people whose dementia is less severe.

Validation therapy aims to reduce negative behaviors by empathizing with the emotional content of patients' experiences. It's different from reality orientation in that it's concerned more with underlying feelings than with accurate current perception.

Problem adaptation therapy tries to reduce depression by working with families and others to redirect patients' attention away from situations that cause sadness and give them more positive ways of looking at reality.

Behavioral approaches try to reduce disruptive behaviors by periodically rewarding patients for not engaging in them.

Although it's not technically a form of therapy, a technique called *environmental intervention* is based on the idea that since people with dementia no longer have the ability to adapt to their environment, the environment should be adapted to them. It tries to create surroundings that are safe, stress free, and comfortable, and provide a familiar daily schedule that varies as little as possible so as to reduce disorientation.

Do these approaches work? Yes, sometimes. There's conflicting evidence, but a lot of studies have shown that they can have a positive impact on patients' quality of life.

What about MCI?

Apart from Aduhelm, there are no drugs on the market that have been approved for MCI, although there is some evidence that taking melatonin at night can improve cognitive functioning in people with MCI.

Most doctors recommend that patients with MCI adopt healthy lifestyle habits in an effort to improve brain functioning and prevent MCI from developing into full-blown dementia. These habits include exercising regularly, quitting smoking, eating a healthy diet (including fresh fruits and vegetables, whole grains, and lean proteins), and participating in mentally stimulating tasks and social activities. Of course these habits will help anyone to maintain healthy brain functioning as they get older, not just patients with MCI.

II

Understanding Your New Relationship with Your Parent

6

Why Caring for Parents with Dementia Is So Much Harder than Caring for Parents with Other Diseases

Taking care of a parent with a serious disease is always difficult—in addition to the sadness and loss caused by the disease itself, there are a great many physical, emotional, and financial burdens. Nevertheless dementia is different. It's not like other "normal" diseases. And the strain on an adult child trying to take care of a parent with dementia is unique.

It's important to understand why this is so, because understanding the reasons that dementia care is so difficult can go a long way toward helping you to cope with how hard it is.

Here's a look at some of the reasons caring for a parent with dementia is not just difficult, but *much more difficult* than caring for a parent with another type of illness.

Dementia Is Lengthy

A person with dementia can live for many years after a diagnosis. This fact means that children are not just called on to take care of their parents for a few weeks or months, as might be the case with other terminal illnesses. Many children might be able to handle a sprint—they can take time off from work and take on difficult duties, knowing that the change to their lives won't be permanent. But dementia can be a marathon. Children are asked to make major changes in their lives with no end in sight.

A study by the Alzheimer's Association found that 71 percent of family members who care for someone with dementia do so for more than a year, and about a third—32 percent—provide care for more than 5 years.

If a parent lives for a long time, the cumulative effect of caring for someone for years can be overwhelming. And children can easily become hopeless, knowing that their situation isn't a temporary alteration but is likely to go on indefinitely—with no possibility of the parent getting better, and in fact with the certainty that his or her condition will gradually become more and more difficult to handle.

Dementia Is Also Acute

As dementia progresses, the amount of work a son or daughter has to do becomes very significant. The Alzheimer's Association study found that 61 percent of family members of people with dementia provide what is considered to be the highest, most difficult level of care—compared to only 46 percent of people who care for a family member with another serious illness. In addition family members devote more time per week than people caring for someone with a different serious illness. In fact nearly a quarter of family members spend 40 or more hours a week providing care.

The study also found that 49 percent of family members provide financial assistance, amounting on average to hundreds of dollars a month, and that 52 percent have made physical alterations to their own home or to another family member's home.

This combination of a lengthy and acute disease is unusual. For example, many people die of complications of heart disease or diabetes, and these are lengthy diseases, but they don't typically require years of acute care. On the other hand, people in the terminal stages of cancer often require acute care, but this period usually lasts a matter of weeks or months, not years.

Another consideration is that by the time people with other serious illnesses reach the point of needing acute care, they often have medical conditions that require being in a hospital or nursing home, such that much of the care is provided by medically trained staff rather than by family members. Dementia is very unusual in that sufferers often need full-time care, but it's the kind of care that a person without any medical training is able to provide.

The effects of this acute-but-lengthy combination on family members are significant. For instance, the Alzheimer's Association study found that 55 percent of caregivers spend less time with family and friends; 49 percent have sacrificed vacations, hobbies, and social activities; 30 percent have stopped exercising; 18 percent say their health is worse; and 41 percent rate their stress as a 4 or a 5 on a 5-point scale (where 5 is the most stressed). All these findings are worse for people taking care of someone with dementia than for people taking care of someone with another serious illness.

Parents May Be in Denial

Many people in the early stages of dementia are in denial. They don't want to acknowledge (to themselves or to others) that they are having trouble with the tasks of daily life. They insist that they can handle them, and they find ways to cover up their deficits or make excuses for them. The result is that they often make mistakes or do something dangerous but refuse to admit it.

A parent who is in denial creates enormous problems for a care provider.

Take, for example, a parent who is having trouble handling finances. A simple solution might be to set up a joint checking account and for you to take over paying the bills. If your parent were suffering from a different type of serious illness, doing so might be fairly easy and straightforward. Parents who are in denial, however, may object strongly to this arrangement. They may insist that they can handle their finances. They might act suspicious of their child's motives, either because of dementia-related paranoia or simply in an attempt to get the child to back off. And this behavior might continue even as the parent fails to pay bills, pays the wrong amount, forgets about other important financial obligations, or generally makes bad decisions about money.

This is incredibly frustrating. If all you had to do was handle your parent's finances, it would be a burden but it would be manageable. Instead children of dementia sufferers often end up having to constantly remind their parents of tasks that need to be done, and then check later to see if they were. They seem to continually discover—too late!—that their parent failed to do something and, instead of just being able to do it themselves, they have to go to great lengths to undo the resulting mess. They are constantly playing catch-up.

And that's just finances! Similar problems arise in a lot of other areas as well, from taking care of a house to prescriptions and medical appointments.

A common refrain of family members is "It would be easy if all I had to do was take care of her, instead of constantly dealing with her trying to take care of herself!" And this is a problem that largely doesn't exist with other types of serious illness.

Parents May Not Understand Their Own Limitations

Not all the problems described in the last section are the result of denial. It's also the case that, because the disease makes it hard to understand things, parents often simply don't comprehend that they have lost the ability to handle important matters.

For instance, if parents forget to pay a bill, they might not immediately notice. When mailings start to arrive about the missed payment, they might not understand them, or they might mistakenly think that the problem has already been taken care of. Even if they realize that they made a mistake, they might promptly forget that they did—or that they made a number of other similar mistakes recently.

As a result, when their children suggest that they need help with their finances, they might be genuinely bewildered (or offended) at the suggestion.

Parents May Not Understand Your Help

When parents have a different serious illness and their children have to help them with something—say, giving them a bath—the parents might be angry or frustrated about being unable to do it by themselves, but they at least understand that their child is helping them take a bath. They are more likely to cooperate and assist the child to whatever extent they're able.

But parents with advanced dementia are often unable to understand what's happening to them. They might be unwilling to get undressed or even become terrified of the water. They might have no understanding that the child is attending to their personal hygiene and become agitated or hostile. At the very least, they will have little ability to cooperate with the process and make it easier for the child.

And this is true not just with regard to giving someone a bath. Countless other daily activities—getting parents dressed, getting them to eat a meal, cleaning their dentures, or getting them to a medical appointment—can become a major struggle.

This in itself is a huge difference between taking care of someone with dementia and taking care of someone with a different type of illness. It's one thing to take care of someone's personal hygiene and assist with other daily activities; it's another thing altogether when doing so can result at any time in an unpleasant scene or a battle of wills.

Some parents with dementia will only occasionally become agitated by attempts to help them. Nevertheless the fact that the child knows that the parent *might* become agitated is itself a source of constant stress. And even if the parent doesn't become upset, the fact that the parent doesn't understand what the child is doing and is unable to cooperate— or has to be cajoled into cooperating—makes the burden much worse than it is for someone who is taking care of a parent with a different disease.

You May Feel Guilty

Because parents often can't understand or cooperate with their adult children's attempts to help them, the children can end up feeling guilty. Of course, they are merely trying to help their parents accomplish a necessary task, but it's hard not to feel guilty when the result is that parents become upset, scared, or miserable.

In addition some parents with dementia also become paranoid. They may accuse their children of trying to hurt them, of stealing from them, and so on. These accusations are obviously not true, but being accused of harming a parent can still make children feel considerable grief. And this is yet another burden that children whose parents have a different illness don't generally have to deal with.

Guilt feelings can arise from other issues too. Some children feel guilty because they believe that they are in effect reversing the roles— suddenly treating their parent more like a child. Some feel guilty because, in their frustration, they end up getting angry at a parent. And some feel guilty because in certain situations the easiest course of action is to lie to or mislead the parent.

Children may also feel guilty because they sometimes have to make decisions for their parents that are different from what the parents, in their diminished mental state, currently say they want. For instance, some parents will plead with their children, "Promise me you'll never put me into one of those homes!" This can be difficult because the child may know that at some point the parent will need round-the-clock medical care.

A related problem is that spending a lot of time with a parent, combined with the stress and frustration of dealing with the disease, can sometimes cause a grown child who has previously established a healthy adult relationship with a parent—and who no longer has that same relationship due to the illness—to fall back into older and less constructive emotional patterns, such as those that existed when the child was a teenager. This situation can also lead to feelings of guilt.

Other Family Members May Be in Denial

People in the early stages of dementia aren't the only ones who can be in denial about the disease. Many family members are also in denial. They may be psychologically unready to admit that a loved one has a serious and ultimately terminal illness. They might not want to think about how much work will be involved in taking care of the person. They might also be afraid of how the loved one will react if they start being honest about the problem.

Of course denial isn't the only reason that family members may be unable to acknowledge dementia. The fact that the disease develops so gradually and that the symptoms sometimes resemble normal aging can simply make it hard to perceive.

Perhaps you've had an experience in which someone who hasn't seen your children for a year exclaims, "My, how they've grown!" The fact that the person hasn't seen your children for a while means that they're comparing their memory to the present reality and noticing the difference. Parents, on the other hand, see their children every day, and the difference each day is so small that it's hard to notice. In the same way, adult children who don't see their parent every day may have an easier time picking up the signs of dementia. A spouse, sibling, or other person who sees the parent very regularly may have a harder time noticing the development of the disease simply because the changes each day are relatively minimal.

One problem with family-member denial is that two people who are both in denial tend to reinforce each other. It's easier for people who have early dementia to deny this fact if their spouse is also denying it, and vice versa.

Family-member denial can make it much harder to take care of a parent with dementia. For instance, you might be unable to get family members' help in dealing with a problem or cooperation in arranging a treatment. Family members might also block your steps to arrange the parent's finances in a way that will prevent problems down the road. Sometimes denial can lead to serious friction between family members. There have been cases in which a child is trying to help a parent and the child's siblings make accusations that the child is exaggerating symptoms, promoting dependence, being bossy, or seeking undue control over the parent's finances.

Of course family-member denial isn't unique to dementia. It can exist with other illnesses. But it tends to be more prevalent with dementia because in the early stages it's easier to hide or explain away the symptoms. Also other diseases tend to result in more clear-cut diagnoses and the need to quickly make treatment choices. The fact that dementia is harder to diagnose and treat makes it easier to keep denying that it's real. So once again, dementia sufferers can become much harder to care for than people with other diseases.

Other People's Lack of Understanding

If you tell someone that you're taking care of a parent with cancer, you're likely to get a lot of sympathy. The other person might not know all the minor details of cancer care, but they will have a general sense that it's a very difficult task. But if you tell someone that you're taking care of a parent with dementia, the reaction is likely to be different. Most people who haven't dealt personally with a dementia sufferer simply have no idea what's involved and can't appreciate the level of work and stress that you're experiencing.

In part that's because dementia is a "hidden" disease. Once dementia reaches a certain point, it's dangerous for people to be out in the community, at least unless someone is guiding them every step of the way. Many people are kept largely at home or in a dedicated facility. But the result of the fact that dementia is largely invisible is that the general public's experience of the disease is usually very limited, perhaps to occasionally seeing a distant relative who has some trouble remembering people's names.

Because the people in your social circle—on whom you usually rely for support—will likely have little if any experience or understanding of what a person with fairly advanced dementia is like, it will probably be very hard for them to express an appropriate level of sympathy. (That's a big reason that support groups for family members are a good idea. You can find more information on such groups in the Resources section.)

Embarrassment

Dementia is a brain disorder. Unlike cancer or kidney disease, it results in symptoms that are not just physical but behavioral. As a result, dementia sufferers can have great difficulty coping with common tasks and always have the potential to do or say something that is socially inappropriate.

Many family members who are taking care of a parent with early dementia want to find outside activities for them, such as going to a park or out to lunch. And certain activities might be necessary, like going to a shoe store or a medical appointment. Yet these situations can result in awkward and embarrassing moments.

A busy waitress, for instance, is unlikely to understand why a parent can't decipher a menu, can't follow a recital of salad dressings, or gets confused when asked if she wants more coffee. A person in a doctor's waiting room is unlikely to understand why your parent keeps mistaking him for a childhood friend. And these are minor problems—sometimes a parent can say or do something that is truly inappropriate, shocking, or humiliating.

Perhaps such embarrassing behaviors occur only rarely. But the fact that they *could* happen at any time causes family members to be constantly on their toes. It's a type of stress that simply doesn't exist for people who are taking care of parents with other illnesses.

Being "Always on Call"

People who are taking care of a parent with a different serious illness are often able to set up a schedule. It's a lot of work, but there are times when the person can simply "unplug" and rest for a while.

But the problem with dementia is that a person who can't tell what time it is simply can't be scheduled. Parents may get up at 3:00 A.M., think it's 3:00 P.M., and need your full attention. In addition it's often impossible to make a schedule because there's no way to know how long a particular task will take. Getting someone dressed might take 2 minutes one day and a half-hour the next—if you can succeed at all.

The result of the chaos, unpredictability, and lack of scheduling is a feeling of being "always on call." You never know when something will go wrong, and you'll have to drop everything and respond to it. This level of stress might be manageable if it were for a limited time, but the fact that dementia is such a lengthy disease means that there is no end to what you will be called upon to do. The resulting feeling that you no longer have any control over your own life is an incredible burden for family members.

The Thankless Task

When grown children take care of parents with a different type of disease, the parents may be frustrated at not being able to take care of themselves, but in most cases they will deeply appreciate what the children are doing and express their gratitude.

Sadly, however, many parents with dementia simply cannot understand everything their children do for them and are too confused to be able to say "thank you." In fact, parents may express opposition to their children's efforts to help them and may be paranoid and suspicious, accusing the child of trying to harm them.

The result is that caring for a parent with dementia is often literally a thankless task.

People are sometimes able to make great sacrifices if they feel that their sacrifices serve an important cause and if they feel that what they do is appreciated. Unfortunately, one of the abilities dementia often robs parents of is the ability to express appreciation.

This feeling of thanklessness can be compounded when friends don't understand how hard you have to work, and it can especially be compounded if siblings or other family members don't understand the work involved—or are in denial and think that what you're doing is unnecessary or selfish.

In some cases of early dementia, the family decides that it's a shameful secret and tries to keep everyone from talking about it to the outside world. If this happens and you don't have people to reach out to for support, the situation can be even more isolating and depressing.

Dementia also robs parents of the ability to express feedback. People who have to do a difficult job are often more motivated if they can get some response indicating how well they're doing it and where they can improve. This gives them a sense of pride, mastery, and satisfaction that makes the task more enjoyable.

With dementia, family members often feel like they're operating in a void. Am I doing a good job? Could I do anything better? The lack of feedback in response to their efforts becomes yet another source of stress.

Complex Grief and Loss

When a loved one dies after a relatively short illness, people generally experience grief. There is an intense period of feeling the loss that typically lasts from 2 to 6 months. The feeling of loss never fully goes away, but after a few months most people regain the ability to go on with their lives.

Many people are helped during this period by two ways in which society responds to the death of a loved one. One is a sudden outpouring of sympathy from family and friends. The other is the rituals that our society has for dealing with death, such as religious services, funeral traditions, sympathy cards, and so on.

But for people taking care of a parent with dementia, it's all far more complicated.

When someone has advanced dementia, the person seems no longer to be there. It can easily feel as though the person has died, and you definitely grieve the loss—the loss of the person and the loss of a joint history and the ability to share memories. And yet the person *hasn't* died. You can't mourn in a natural way because your parent is still here—and still needs to be cared for. There is no sudden outpouring of sympathy from family and friends. There are no rituals or traditions that recognize and support you in this kind of loss. It's like a limbo of grief.

There are two terms that are sometimes used to describe certain complex forms of grieving. One is *ambiguous loss*, which refers to a loss that has no closure. An example would be the experience of the family of a soldier who is missing in combat. The family members feel grief, but they don't have closure because there is no proof that the person has actually died.

Another term is *disenfranchised loss*, which refers to a terrible loss that is not socially recognized or that is hard to talk about publicly. An example is the loss of a much-beloved pet. Many people feel intense grief over the loss of a pet, but they find it hard to express their feelings, because there are no social rituals or traditions that reflect what they're feeling.

Dementia caregivers often experience both types of loss. They no longer have the person they loved, but there is no closure for them because the person hasn't died, and the loss is not one that is socially recognized or that is easy to talk about with other people. The result is that they carry around a unique and difficult emotional burden that they often find impossible to express.

● ● ●

When you read through this list, it's easy to see that caring for a parent with dementia is utterly unlike caring for a parent with most any other type of serious illness. The length and intensity of the disease, the inability of the patient to understand or cooperate with care, the lack of social support, and the many kinds of stresses inherent in providing care can make the problem seem truly overwhelming.

Indeed while many people who don't understand the disease might assume that it's possible to take care of a parent with dementia and retain your own sanity, it's much easier said than done. In order to accomplish the task, it's necessary to have a *strategy*. And that strategy is what this book is designed to give you.

7

The Biggest Mistake
Family Members Make

As seen in the last chapter, caring for a parent with dementia is much more difficult than caring for a parent with a different type of disease. But that difficulty is made much worse by the fact that most family members tend to approach the task in a way that doesn't lead to optimal results, either for themselves or for the dementia sufferer.

There are a number of reasons why this is so. But many of them can be summarized with this observation: *Family members often don't approach dementia as a "real" disease. They don't treat it the same way they would a different type of illness, such as cancer or heart disease.*

When a parent is diagnosed with cancer, for instance, family members may be in shock and initially respond with some denial or avoidance. And yet the clear medical evidence of the problem, the parent's often-significant symptoms, and the need to make difficult decisions about near-term treatment tend to force the family to focus on the issues and on the necessity of making choices about the future. Family members often quickly become realistic about what needs to be done and develop a plan for coping with the disease process.

With dementia, however, it's much easier to put off developing such a plan. There are a number of reasons why this is true.

It's Not as Obvious That It's a Disease. The fact that the symptoms of early dementia sometimes mimic normal aging can make it harder to understand and accept the seriousness of the illness.

The Lack of a Clear-Cut Diagnosis. Because dementia is always a probable diagnosis, with no clear evidence resulting from a medical test, it can seem less real to families. In addition many families never actually get a diagnosis at all, often because the patient doesn't want them to.

The Nature of the Medical System. Unfortunately primary care doctors often have little education or training regarding dementia assessment and treatment. Many of them are uncomfortable with making and communicating a diagnosis and explaining the progression of the disease to family members. And it's not uncommon for them to have difficulty in making referrals to specialists in behavioral neurology or geriatric psychiatry because of a lack of specialty providers.

The Lack of Urgent Symptoms or Patient Complaints. When someone has a heart attack, there's no questioning the seriousness of the situation. Most other diseases announce themselves with significant pain or discomfort. But with dementia, especially early dementia, there are seldom urgent problems that would land someone in an emergency room. The absence of an air of crisis—coupled with the fact that people with the disease may not be fully aware of their own symptoms—can make families less concerned about coming up with a plan.

It's a Lengthy Disease. With many serious illnesses, there's a sense that the patient will only have a certain amount of time to live, at least without treatment or if the treatment is unsuccessful. But the fact that dementia can last for many years creates less of a sense of urgency.

The Lack of Highly Effective Treatment. One of the features that makes cancer and other diseases seem real to families is the need to make quick medical decisions. With dementia, the fact that there are few effective treatments means that the initial experience involves far less rushing and stress. In addition, with a disease that requires quick medical decisions, doctors usually spend a considerable amount of time explaining the illness and what is likely to happen as it progresses so that the patient and family can make informed choices. Because dementia offers fewer choices, families often don't get this kind of detailed information. (Although doctors can help, some are reluctant to discuss the progress of the disease precisely because it means admitting that there are no easy cures.)

Variability. Even if a doctor wants to explain the course of the disease to a family in detail, it can be difficult. The progress of the disease is a lot more variable than that of pancreatic cancer, for example. It's hard to predict exactly what will happen next. This is especially true because it's not always clear whether the person has Alzheimer's disease, Lewy body dementia, or some other form.

It's Not Cared for in a Medical Setting. The reality of someone's having a serious illness is often brought home to families by being in the medical settings where they are cared for—hospitals, doctors' offices, and so on. The fact that dementia sufferers usually receive care at home—and what they receive is more in the nature of tending to personal needs rather than esoteric medical procedures—once again reduces the family's sense of urgency.

It Can Be Easy to Cope at the Beginning. Very early dementia can be relatively easy to deal with. The person with the disease is not in pain and may not yet have significant behavioral problems. The types of care that family members have to provide are fairly simple, which can create a false sense that the problem doesn't require a life-changing amount of work.

The Larger Culture. Movies, television, and other forms of popular culture often dramatize cancer and other serious illnesses. That's because the diseases themselves are often more dramatic, and the characters who experience them can be portrayed without cognitive deficits. Dementia is much more invisible so families have less of an idea of what may be in store.

Stigma. Dementia is stigmatized in our culture, and it's often considered embarrassing to admit it or talk about it, which creates an incentive for families to avoid the subject.

For all these reasons, many families don't develop a sense that dementia is a real disease on a par with other terminal illnesses. It seems profoundly sad, but not like an emergency.

As a result, they don't feel a pressing need to make plans. They adopt a wait-and-see attitude. They "take each day as it comes." In the initial stages, they make minor changes in their life to accommodate the illness, and they figure that they will be able to continue doing so indefinitely.

Why a Delay in Making a Plan Is a Mistake

Imagine a house that needs a new roof. The first sign of a problem is a very minor ceiling leak when it rains. The owner puts a bucket under the leak to catch the few drops of water, then dries and patches the ceiling. This quick fix is a lot easier than replacing the whole roof, he thinks.

Later there's another storm and a slightly bigger leak. Then a storm with two leaks. Then another. Finally the area experiences several weeks of heavy rain. The leaks come one after another. Before the owner can fix one problem, another starts. He spends all his time running around and dealing with the leaks, but he can't keep up with them, let alone do anything else. And while he could replace the roof, he's now so busy dealing with the consequences of not having replaced it that he no longer has the time. He's spending every minute playing a constant game of catch-up . . . and losing.

That's what it's like for families taking care of someone with dementia. A few extra burdens gradually turn into a lot of burdens and then into a constant burden. Family members become exhausted and feel that there just aren't enough hours in the day. They can never catch up or get ahead.

As a care provider, the best thing you can do is to take dementia seriously at the outset as a real disease. This doesn't mean you need to panic, but it means that you need to focus and make a plan for how to cope as the disease progresses. Thinking ahead is the equivalent of replacing the roof. It's not easy, and it takes some work at the beginning, but it will pay enormous dividends in the future.

What "Making a Plan" Means

What does it mean to make a plan for a parent with dementia?

With other diseases, doctors frequently talk in terms of a treatment plan. With cancer, for instance, the plan might involve making choices among possible remedies—radiation, surgery, chemotherapy, and so on. There might be a number of contingencies—if this happens, we'll do this, but if that happens instead, we'll do that. Basically the doctor provides a road map for how to approach the disease.

Although treatment plans can be difficult for family members to contemplate, they're actually enormously helpful to families. Among other things, road maps give family members a sense of orientation and efficacy. They turn a big, scary, amorphous problem into a series of practical steps that can be taken. They put people on the same page and give them a sense of purpose.

Unfortunately because there's so little that the medical establishment can do about dementia, doctors seldom give family members a treatment plan for it. They tend to tell them that the disease will get worse over time and perhaps prescribe a drug or two that might or might not have some limited benefit.

This puts family members in limbo. Because they receive little or no medical guidance, it's natural that they adopt a policy of taking each day as it comes.

But you need a plan for dementia every bit as much as you need a plan for cancer! In fact you probably need one even more, because (as we've seen) the demands on families can be far greater for dementia than for other diseases. And since the medical establishment isn't going to be much help in giving you one, you'll need to do it yourself. You'll need to replace your own roof.

A good plan will give you a sense of orientation, purpose, and efficacy and help you to be proactive in taking care of your parent. A good plan involves four elements:

1. Accepting that your relationship to your parent will be forever changed. Certain things may continue for a time of course, but it's inevitable that the disease will fundamentally alter the nature of the connection between you. Accepting this fact is very difficult, and it's a stumbling block for many people. But it's the reality. To refuse to accept it is to be in denial. And to accept it is actually very constructive, because it allows you to begin looking for what can be positive and loving in your new relationship instead of constantly mourning the passing of the old one. This is healthier for you and far better for your parent as well.

2. Accepting that you will need to take care of yourself as you take care of your mother or father. Once again, this arrangement is both healthier for you and far better for your parent. It can also be a stumbling block for some people, but people who don't make plans about how to care for themselves typically end up running themselves into the ground, which isn't good for anyone.

3. Thinking proactively about the issues your parent will confront and how you will cope with them when they occur. How will you deal with your parent's finances? With your parent continuing to want to drive? How will you get help with personal care and other needs once your parent can no longer do certain tasks? How will you prepare yourself emotionally for times when your parent is confused, combative, delusional, or embarrassing? How will you handle difficult behaviors? How will you know your parent's end-of-life wishes?

4. Thinking about what will happen when you can no longer take care of your parent yourself because your parent requires skilled nursing or round-the-clock care. What options do you have, and how can you choose?

These can be very difficult topics. Dementia is different from other diseases such as cancer because in general you don't *have* to think about these topics right away. And most people don't. But not preparing for them is like not replacing your roof—you'll most likely end up hopeless and overwhelmed, constantly playing catch-up instead of following a plan.

The rest of this book is designed to help you address these issues and formulate a plan. It won't make caring for a parent with dementia easy, but it will make it manageable. You'll preserve your own sanity, and along the way you'll actually provide much better, more thoughtful, and more loving care in your parent's declining years.

8

Your New Relationship with Your Parent

It's very difficult to contemplate the idea that your parent has dementia. No one wants to seriously consider that a parent will gradually lose his or her mental faculties and has an ultimately terminal disease. It's no wonder that so many family members try to put off thinking about it in depth for as long as possible.

One of the few consolations of the disease is the knowledge that, compared to many other serious diseases, dementia is in some ways not so bad. Most people who have dementia tend to live a fairly long time with it. Unlike most diseases, for the most part it doesn't cause a lot of physical pain and discomfort. It doesn't usually require painful and difficult treatments, such as chemotherapy. At least in the earlier stages, most dementia sufferers can be cared for at home. Many people with dementia are able to enjoy a reasonably good quality of life for a long time. And while they may gradually lose their mental abilities, most people are able to continue to experience loving emotional relationships for the rest of their lives.

The sad truth is that many adult children are so upset by the losses wrought by dementia that they don't make a concerted effort to maximize the quality of life—their own and that of their parents—that may still be very possible for years to come.

A Different Way to Interact

The most important thing to understand about having a parent with dementia is that *you now have a new relationship with your parent*. Going forward, you will be less and less able to interact with your parent in the way that you did in the past. Your relationship will be very different. And while it's natural to mourn the loss of the person you knew and the relationship you had before, it's also very important to embrace this new relationship. By learning a different way to interact with your parent, you'll be able as far as possible to make your new relationship a loving and rewarding one for you both.

One of the reasons it's difficult to embrace this new relationship is that it's hard to define. It's literally unlike any other relationship in life, so there's no model for it in people's experience.

Because people with dementia sometimes behave in ways that seem childlike (or even childish), it can be tempting to think that taking care of a parent with dementia is like taking care of a child. In general this is a mistake. It may be true that certain experiences one has had in raising children—especially loving them in spite of their foibles and mistakes—can occasionally come in handy. But it can't be emphasized enough that people with dementia are not children; they're adults with a disease process. To treat them as children is to infantilize them. It's also wrong and counterproductive. People with dementia may have memory problems, but they still have adult personalities and they still have a lifetime of lived experience. They can usually sense when they're being treated in a condescending way, and they will likely react negatively to it, if not immediately then eventually. And thinking of your parent as a child negates the actual complex nature of the relationship you can still have.

Relating to a parent with dementia is not like relating to a well parent or a child or anyone else. It's its own experience. The good news is that you can establish the relationship in a way that's creative and healthy or at least as healthy and constructive as possible.

Setting Goals for Your Relationship

Once you accept that you have a new relationship with your parent, the next step is to establish goals for that relationship. This may sound like a strange exercise. After all most people don't think of themselves as going around explicitly creating goals for their relationships with other people.

But in fact in the most important relationships in our lives, we often articulate our goals. In the traditional wedding vows, for instance, couples promise (in various wordings) to love, honor, cherish, and be faithful to each other. Other promises are made in employment contracts and handbooks, in the Hippocratic oath sometimes taken by doctors, in the fiduciary obligations assumed by trustees, and in promises associated with baptisms.

Another way to describe these goals is to see them as *values*. They are the lodestar we look to in order to answer questions about what choices to make in difficult situations.

It might seem odd and pointless to write down your values and goals regarding taking care of a parent with dementia. But putting them on paper is actually one of the most helpful activities you can do. Why? Because with dementia, difficult situations arise all the time—sometimes on a daily basis.

The reality of dementia is that you are constantly confronted with problems to which there is no clear solution. Is it safe for your mother to keep driving? What should you do if your father insists on managing his own medications but you don't trust him to do it correctly? When is antipsychotic medication appropriate? Should you move your parent to a memory-care facility? When? Should you respond to a worried parent's call at 3:00 A.M. if you have to work the next day? Is it okay to lie to parents to get them to do something important? And so on, and on, and on.

One of the most terrible aspects of having a parent with dementia is continually having to make decisions when there is no obvious correct choice and then worrying about whether you did the right thing. This problem is often made worse by the fact that siblings and others may have differing views—or be willing to blame you if you make a particular decision and in retrospect it didn't work out well.

This is why it's helpful to have a clear set of goals. When you're confronted by a difficult decision, you can ask which choice is most in keeping with your objectives. Of course this doesn't mean you'll always be a perfect decision maker, but it does make it easier to avoid agonizing over dilemmas and constantly second-guessing yourself.

The other benefit of having a clear set of goals is that it makes it much easier to be proactive in making some decisions now that will make your and your parent's life easier later. For instance there are many legal and financial steps you can take during early dementia to avoid later problems, and it's helpful in taking these steps to clearly define what your legal and financial objectives are. And if you give some thought early on to questions such as under what conditions you would be willing to move your parent to a care facility or what choices you would make at the end of life—difficult as it is—you'll be much better prepared when you're eventually faced with these decisions.

Dementia tends to confront you with a series of crises—again and again, you're forced to react and make a hard choice with very little warning. Many family members are panicked as a result because they haven't prepared for these decisions, and they don't have a good way of choosing between difficult alternatives. That's why it's so important to start thinking about your goals and values, so you can be as ready as possible when issues arise and not be full of regret and self-recrimination later.

What Are Your Goals?

Most people who sit down to make a list of their goals might start out with something like this:

- I want my parent to be safe.

- I want my parent to be happy.

- I want my parent to be comfortable.

- I want my parent's personal needs to be taken care of.

- I want my parent to stay at home as long as possible.

This certainly sounds like a fine list of goals, doesn't it? But the reality is that there are a lot of problems with it.

For one thing, if you start out with this kind of list, you'll very quickly discover that in the real world these goals often conflict with each other. For instance taking away your mother's car keys might keep her safe, but it might also make her very unhappy. Forcing your father to take a bath against his will means that his personal needs will be taken care of, but he'll be very uncomfortable. Keeping your mother at home as long as possible when she is at risk of falling means that she won't be safe. And so on.

There are other problems with these goals too. One is that they set you up for failure. It's in the nature of dementia that your parent will *inevitably* be unhappy a significant amount of the time. But if your goal is for your parent to be happy, does that mean that you haven't succeeded?

Also these goals don't take your own situation into account. You have your own life, and while you're taking care of your parent you have a lot of other responsibilities that are also important. If your goals are for your parent to be happy and comfortable and remain at home, how do you balance these goals against your own needs and your other responsibilities—because inevitably the two will come into conflict?

What Makes for a Good Goal?

The problem with the types of goals we've just listed is that they're little more than vague aspirations. You can want all of them for your parent—and of course you should—but the truth is that you will often be unable to make them happen. These goals don't help you to make difficult *decisions*—the kind of decisions in which two or more good choices are opposed to each other and you have to choose between them or two or more bad choices are in conflict and you have to decide which one is the least bad.

So that's the first criterion for a good goal—it's something that will guide you in making decisions.

A second criterion for a good goal is that it's something you can do yourself. After all you can only control your own actions, not other people's. A problem with goals such as "I want my parent to be happy" is that it's not a goal for your own behavior; it's a goal for how you want another person to feel. And try as you might, you can't actually control how someone else feels—especially when that person's feelings and cognition are being distorted by a ravaging brain disease.

A final criterion for a good goal is that it's something that's likely to bring you peace and satisfaction, at least in the long term. Caring for someone with dementia can be so difficult and stressful that it's seldom possible to feel a lot of happiness in the moment. So it's sometimes a good idea to imagine yourself many years in the future, looking back in time and reflecting on your last years with your parent. You probably won't remember all the minor day-to-day struggles, but ideally you'll think fondly of moments of emotional closeness when the two of you had a special unspoken bond. Thus a good goal is one that will tend to maximize the kinds of memories you'll want to have years later.

Five Goals That Are Truly Helpful

What follows are five goals that meet these criteria. That's not to say that you have to adopt these goals, but they make for a very good way of thinking realistically and constructively about caring for a parent.

1. WHAT'S MOST IMPORTANT?

For many people, a good goal is to keep asking "What's the most important thing?"

This goal sounds simple, but in the onslaught of responsibilities that come with caring for someone with dementia, it's easy to forget to prioritize and think about what's most important.

A focus on what is most important as a goal can help you make a lot of decisions. For instance, you might be considering having an aide come occasionally to help your parent with bathing, taking medications, and other tasks. Your parent might not be happy about the idea. On the other hand, the aide might free you up to engage in other forms of quality time with your parent, such as holding hands, reminiscing, or engaging in fun activities. Asking yourself what's truly most important can help you make a decision that you'll feel satisfied with rather than guilty about.

Asking "What's the most important thing?" can also help you to focus on the larger picture and not become stressed about issues that you're likely to look back on later as trivial. For instance, suppose your mother is generally happy at a memory-care facility, but the staff manage to misplace one of her sweaters that has sentimental value for you. It's easy to become very upset about this . . . even though your mother probably no longer has the ability to remember that the sweater is missing. Reflecting on what's most important might cause you to decide that the fact that your mother is receiving good care from the staff is more important than the sweater.

Another advantage of asking "What's the most important thing?" is that it helps you remember that you can't do everything. On a given day, your father's closet and dressers might need to be organized, he might need some items from a store, he might need help with laundry, and he might want you to talk with him. It's very easy to end up feeling exhausted from trying to do everything, or to feel guilty because you didn't do everything or you did everything in a slapdash way. Stopping to ask, "What's the most important thing?" reminds you to prioritize, so you can take care of your father's most important needs first and leave things that aren't as urgent for another time.

As the disease progresses, the habit of asking "What's most important?" can help you make wrenching health care decisions. You may have to choose between something that will give your parent comfort and dignity and something else that is likely to prolong his or her life. There are never easy answers to these questions, but being in the habit of asking what's truly most important will allow you to address these dilemmas with much more peace and self-assurance.

Of course it might not always be immediately obvious which of the two choices is the most important. One way to approach this problem is to ask, "If for just a moment my parent could be well and understand everything that I do now, what would he or she want me to do?"

2. FEELINGS, NOT WORDS

Another good goal is "I'll listen to my parent's feelings, not just words."

Communicating with words of course is a major problem for people with dementia. Trouble with language is a hallmark of the disease. For this reason, responding directly to a dementia sufferer's words is not always the best way to interact with the person, and it becomes increasingly true as the illness progresses.

However, dementia sufferers continue to have feelings and emotions. These feelings may be very much affected by the frustration of being unable to communicate with words, but on the other hand, they become even more important because they become the primary way that dementia sufferers *do* communicate with others.

As a result people who take care of someone with dementia need to learn a new language—the language of feelings—or at least they need to begin using that language in a more holistic and deliberate way than they have in the past.

For example, your father might try to tell you something, but be unable to find the words necessary to express the thought. If you focus too hard on trying to decipher the meaning, it's likely that both of you will end up frustrated. But even if you can't figure out his exact meaning, you can probably tell if he's trying to say something that's happy, sad, or amusing. By mirroring his emotions, you can at least express that he has communicated what he's feeling—which may in the end be more important than the precise sentence he had in mind.

Or perhaps your mother will tell you something that's clearly not true, such as that tomorrow is her birthday or that she got a phone call from a long-dead relative. You could try to respond to her words on a literal level, in which case you would end up contradicting her and perhaps making her sad or argumentative. Or, rather than responding to her words, you could simply respond to her feelings. "You seem very happy about that. That's wonderful!" you might say. By responding in this way, you haven't actually agreed that your mother received a phone call from a dead person, but you've validated what she's feeling and shared her happiness.

People with dementia often become frustrated because they can't express their needs. At the root of a great deal of dementia-related anger and behavioral problems is an unmet need that ends up getting expressed in a twisted way through stubbornness, accusations, and so on.

Of course when people become angry with us, we have a natural tendency to become defensive. If our parents accuse us of stealing money or not caring about them (despite all the work we've done), it's natural to take offense and verbally defend ourselves. However, what we're really doing in such situations is responding to words and not to feelings. A better approach is almost always to acknowledge the parent's feelings ("I'm very sorry that you're so upset") and then try to understand what's really causing the unhappiness. It's hard to ignore someone who is accusing you of something you didn't do, but having adopted an explicit goal of focusing on feelings and not just words can be a big help.

By the way, these first two goals are often also seen in healthy marital relationships. Almost all couples fight. But partners who are good at defusing fights are those who can set aside the other's hurtful words, acknowledge the other's feelings, and try to understand the person's deeper motivations. They also tend to be able to resolve disagreements by focusing on what is most important rather than on trying to win every small battle.

3. FIXING AND SYMPATHIZING

Another good goal is "I'll fix what I can, and as for what I can't, I'll sympathize."

One of the reasons that taking care of a parent with dementia is so difficult is that so many problems that arise are ones that you can't do anything about. Your parent is unhappy about the situation, but there's nothing you can do to solve the problem.

Feeling helpless can leave you feeling like a failure—especially if one of your goals is "I want my parent to be happy."

The advantage of saying "I'll fix it if I can" is that it explicitly acknowledges that there are many problems that you *can't* fix. You don't have to feel guilty because you can't work miracles. Also it gives you something you *can* do if you can't make the problem go away. Sympathy might not seem like much, but it's often the best you can do, and frequently it's very much appreciated by parents because it at least signals that you understand what they're going through.

Having this as a goal can help you make decisions in situations where parents are scared, angry, or suspicious about something that is important for them. For instance, parents might be afraid or upset about going to the dentist because they can't fully understand what's happening to them, and you can't entirely remove the frightening nature of it, but you can often be a tremendous help just by acknowledging that going to the dentist can be upsetting or scary and sympathizing with your parent's feelings.

This is one case where there are certain parallels with raising a small child. Small children might be upset about going to the doctor or getting a vaccination because they live in the present and they haven't yet mastered the idea of enduring something unpleasant now in order to prevent something much more harmful later. A parent can't fix this problem. Giving in to the child and not getting a vaccine is out of the question, but being mad at the child for resisting will only make things worse. The best approach is to insist on going to the doctor but express sympathy for how unpleasant it is for the child.

Of course sympathy isn't magic and doesn't always work. Your parent might still get upset and act out. But at least you know that you've done everything you can, so you don't need to feel guilty.

This goal can also be a helpful response to the fact that many people with dementia feel depressed. It's very natural to feel depressed; almost anyone would feel sad and helpless about the loss of memory and cognition. You can't just make your parent's depression go away, no matter how much you want to, but you can express sympathy. Just saying "This must be hard for you" at least reassures your parent that you understand what he or she is experiencing.

Interestingly "I'll fix what I can, and as for what I can't, I'll sympathize" is an important attitude for yourself as well. You can't always "fix" your parent, and when you can't, you should sympathize with yourself, rather than blaming yourself for something that's not your fault. After all the true culprit is a disease over which no one has any control.

4. THE "GOOD ENOUGH" RELATIONSHIP

A fourth goal is "I will work to have a *good enough* relationship with my parent."

Dementia can be extremely sad because you lose the relationship you once had with your mother or father. If you were close and happy, you'll find that a lot of that closeness may change—after all, you have a new relationship. Many people become caught up in mourning the loss of the way they used to get along with their parent. They think more about what's missing than about what they still have.

Another problem is that it always seems like there is no end to all that you *could* be doing for your parent. Caring for a parent is not a discrete task like washing the dishes, in which there comes a point where everything is clean and put away and you're finished. When caring for someone with dementia, you're never finished, and there is always more you could do. As a result, many people feel guilty because they don't live up to an ideal in their head of what they could or should be doing—or what they think their parent needs them to do.

The goal of working toward a "good enough" relationship helps with both these problems. It does so because it requires an acknowledgment that there is no perfect relationship and that the kind of relationship you had before is no longer possible because of the disease. What *is* possible is a good enough relationship—one in which you care well enough for your parent and you're as close as you can be given the circumstances.

Training yourself to ask "Is what I'm doing good enough?" rather than "Have I done everything I possibly can?" will allow you to act more reasonably and feel happier about the efforts you've made. Asking "Is my relationship good enough?" will encourage you to focus on the relationship you still can have with your parent, rather than thinking solely of what you have lost.

5. RESPECTING YOUR OWN BOUNDARIES

A final goal to consider is "I will respect my own boundaries."

We all have a lot of responsibilities in life, and we create boundaries in order to make it possible to meet those responsibilities. For instance, while it might be fun to stay out all night, we try to go to bed at a reasonable hour if we know we need to get up early the next morning. We try to be responsible for our health by eating well and exercising. We might work hard, but we don't work so hard that we have no time left for our family, social life, or recreation.

We may love our family and friends, but we expect that they won't place so many demands on us that we won't be able to handle our other responsibilities. And for the most part, family and friends do respect our boundaries in this way.

The problem is that, when a parent develops dementia, respect for boundaries tends to go out the window.

There are two reasons for this. One is that people who suffer from dementia typically require an extraordinary amount of care. At a certain point, there is literally no end to the amount of help that could be given them. As a result, without intending to, a parent may have needs that simply cannot be met without the family member giving up the ability to handle other important responsibilities.

The other reason is that the cognitive problems caused by dementia usually result in parents losing their ability to understand that their adult children have boundaries. They simply don't comprehend that they can't spend all their time with them or can't deal with everything they need. They may forget that their son or daughter has a job or a family or doesn't live with them. If they're awake at 3:00 A.M., it might not occur to them that it's not a good time to call on the phone.

It's obvious—at least if you're not in the middle of the situation—that a person who doesn't have any boundaries is going to become overwhelmed and will ultimately be *less* able to take good care of the parent. That's why respecting your own boundaries is a good goal, albeit one that's easier said than accomplished.

This goal can help you make some tough decisions. For instance, suppose your parent is unhappy about the idea of having an aide come occasionally to help with care, but you're exhausted from trying to do everything yourself. Although your parent might resist getting help from an aide, the goal of respecting your boundaries means that you also have to consider the other side of the equation. If you become short-tempered, irritable, and unhealthy because you're at your wits' end, you're going to provide *worse* care—whether your parent is able to realize it or not. So you might conclude that the aide will actually benefit both of you.

Respecting your own boundaries is part of the larger project of caring for your own needs, which is discussed more in Chapter 10.

The five goals outlined here—asking what's most important, focusing on feelings, sympathizing with what you can't fix, aiming for a "good enough" relationship, and respecting your own boundaries—are very helpful guideposts throughout the process of caring for a parent with dementia. They can help you feel calmer, make better decisions, and approach everything you do with more confidence—in other words, to care smarter. Of course you may want to think about other goals or values too. But whatever you decide, having a sense of what you want to accomplish in caring for your parent is far better than "taking it as it comes," which is a synonym for being unprepared and always reacting in a panic to a crisis.

After all, as Yogi Berra once said, "If you don't know where you're going, you'll end up somewhere else!"

9

Your Relationship with Your Other Parent or Stepparent

In families of a parent with dementia, roughly half the time there's another parent or stepparent in the picture. Usually this parent or stepparent steps in and takes over the bulk of the person's care. You might assume that this situation makes adult children's lives much easier, and it usually does . . . at least at first.

The problem, though, is that as the disease progresses the well spouse almost always reaches a point where it's no longer possible to handle the strain. It becomes too much for one person to bear. And when this occurs, it's extremely common for such spouses to be very reluctant to admit what's happening and to bring in outside help.

This reaction of the well spouse can create a gut-wrenching problem for a son or daughter. You might perceive that your well parent isn't able to provide all the care that your other parent needs and that your other parent is suffering unnecessarily as a result . . . and yet it's very difficult to do anything about it because your well parent seems to be in charge and isn't acknowledging the problem. You might also perceive that your well parent is buckling under the pressure and is also suffering unnecessarily, but won't accept any assistance. As a result, you now have two "problem parents" to deal with instead of one.

While this issue doesn't arise in every single family, it's extremely common. This chapter discusses how to deal with this situation. If you're facing this kind of problem, the sad truth is that you don't just need to develop a new relationship with your parent who has dementia; you also need in some way to develop a new relationship with your parent who *doesn't* have the disease.

The Other Spouse's Denial

The first point to keep in mind is that when a spouse develops dementia, the other spouse almost always experiences some degree of denial. Perhaps there are a few spouses who are completely clear-eyed about the disease process, but they're extreme outliers. Almost always it's not a question of whether a spouse will be in denial; it's just a question of degree.

Common symptoms of denial include not honestly admitting how bad things are, acting like the person's best days are the norm, and being unwilling to acknowledge or discuss the fact that dementia is a progressive disease and will get much worse over time.

Of course "denial" is a tricky term and it's easy to misuse it. Some children will say that their parent is in denial when in fact there's just a legitimate disagreement over how to interpret symptoms or the type of care that's appropriate. Couples have a right to choose their lifestyle, and while their adult children may believe that their parents' home life is too disorderly or that one parent is working too hard, these are decisions that parents are entitled to make.

The problem occurs when well spouses are genuinely endangering their own health and/or failing to provide truly necessary care to the other spouse. Sometimes talking to a professional can help you decide if you simply have different perspectives and opinions from your well parent or if your parents are actually in trouble.

Also, as described in Chapter 1, a certain amount of denial can be healthy. Denial exists to protect us from experiences that would otherwise be a terrible shock to our psychological and emotional well-being and to allow us to come to terms with traumatic situations gradually rather than in a sudden and debilitating way. Again the problem occurs at the point where denial isn't just helping to ease the suffering but is in fact creating additional suffering.

There are a number of reasons well parents may be in denial, but a big one is grief. There are few life events more traumatic than losing a spouse; it's generally a loss of the person you're closest to in life, whom you trust more than anyone else, and whom you rely on for security and comfort. And dementia definitely means that you're losing that person, just in a gradual way. Most people have great difficulty recognizing, accepting, and processing such a loss. And the fact that the disease is gradual means that denial is much easier, because it's possible not to recognize it for a long time and to continue acting like everything will be okay.

Sometimes spouses are in denial not just because they feel grief, but because they literally can't perceive how difficult day-to-day life has become. If you live with someone every day, it can be easy not to notice a gradual decline. Each day you make a small accommodation and it doesn't seem like much, but over time the small accommodations add up to enormous changes in lifestyle. The spouse adjusts to an escalating "new normal" without perceiving just how new and different it is. It's like the fable of the boiling frog; the frog is put in tepid water that is slowly heated and it doesn't notice the gradual change before it's boiled alive.

It's also the case that sometimes spouses are unable to perceive a dementia sufferer's decline because they are experiencing very early dementia symptoms themselves.

Many spouses don't want to admit the degree of difficulty they're living with because they feel a need to protect their adult children. They don't want them to see how badly their other parent is doing, and they don't want them to worry about them and how hard their life has become. They might also not want to be thought of as weak or incompetent.

A final problem is that many spouses develop the idea that caring for their sick spouse is their mission in life. It becomes their job and a measure of their success as a person. They end up believing that any acknowledgment that they can't handle this new normal or that their loved one needs more care than they can provide is an admission of failure on their part. Admitting that they're not up to the task makes them feel helpless and worthless. Their attitude is that, even if caring for their spouse kills them, they have a duty to "go down with the ship."

The underlying reason for this problem usually involves a loss of identity. Well spouses may have spent many years thinking of themselves as the family provider or caretaker, and the idea of no longer being able to fulfill that role makes them feel as though they don't know who they are anymore and have no reason to live.

The feeling of being a failure is incredibly common. As with denial, it's usually not a question of whether a well spouse will feel this way; it's a question of degree. Some spouses are quite willing to accept small amounts of help. Often the sticking point occurs when it becomes necessary to bring in an outside care provider or transition the spouse with dementia to a care facility, because these steps make it clear that there is now a "real" problem. Many well spouses will go to great lengths to avoid these steps, no matter how obvious it becomes that they're necessary, because it seems to them like an admission that they have failed.

Many well spouses in this situation will insist that they need to be the sole caregiver because that's what the other spouse would want. Of course there's often a certain amount of psychological projection in this attitude. It's not at all clear that spouses with dementia would want inadequate care provided by loved ones who are harming their own health. Well spouses may be projecting their own wants onto the other spouse.

Although every family is different, statistically women tend to wait longer than men before seeking outside help. They're more likely to provide extensive personal care and try to handle complex behavioral problems on their own. It's not clear why this is the case, though, and financial as well as emotional reasons might be responsible.

There's also a generational element. Many elderly people grew up at a time when family members lived nearby and took care of older relatives as a matter of course. Their adult children's generation might be much more comfortable taking advantage of the growing personal-care service industry.

There may be cultural factors at work as well. Different nationalities may have different expectations regarding family caregiving, which can influence how willing a well spouse is to ask for help (and sometimes which family members are asked for help).

How Well Spouses Behave

The most common result of a well spouse being in denial is that he or she refuses to acknowledge the true condition of the spouse with dementia and becomes overwhelmed and miserable but doesn't admit it.

This kind of denial can be incredibly frustrating to children, who often have a sense that their parent with dementia is doing badly but can't talk openly about it or get necessary information about his or her condition. Worse, they may perceive that the parent with dementia needs more care—such as going to medical appointments, help with bathing, stimulation, healthier meals, and so on—and isn't receiving it because the well spouse isn't being honest about the situation.

When a child asks questions about the parent with dementia, many well spouses give cryptic responses that leave the child struggling to read between the lines. This can lead to gnawing frustration, guilt, and worry with no good way to handle it.

A very common scenario is that the well spouse keeps insisting that everything is fine, and then suddenly calls the child in a crisis. "Your mom is in the hospital," the father will say; "can you come stay here for a few days?" Then he or she will drop everything and respond. Once the crisis is over, the child will go back to getting no real information until it's necessary to suddenly upend all of life again for the next crisis. This results in a counterproductive cycle in which steps that could help both spouses are never taken and the child ends up being on call at all times and experiencing major unplanned-for disruptions in work, family life, and emotional well-being.

Some parents sincerely want their children to help but find it impossible to admit it. As a result, they behave in ways that are designed to elicit help but pressure them into not acknowledging the situation or the fact that they are providing assistance. Such behavior can be extremely frustrating for the child because it makes it a lot harder to provide help, and it also means that he or she gets no appreciation for what are often very significant sacrifices and efforts at being supportive.

Some parents who are experiencing a great deal of frustration and helplessness behave in ways that are designed to make their children also feel frustrated and helpless. They don't do this because they're mean; they do it because they don't know how to handle their emotions, and it makes them feel better if they can cause someone else to experience something akin to what they're going through.

Some parents simply shut their children out and refuse to let them help at all.

Finally, some parents are aware of their feelings and frustrations but use their child as a therapist. They call their child and tell him in great detail how much they're suffering. This can be helpful to the parent, but it can also be incredibly emotionally draining for the child who is already worried about the parent with dementia and now has to be on call to provide extensive psychological support to the well spouse too.

How Children React

Sometimes children are also in denial. However, it's far more common for them to have a more clear-eyed view of their parent's condition and prognosis than the well spouse does.

Children react to this situation in different ways. Frustration and anger are very common. These feelings can be corrosive because you can't deal with them directly by confronting the well spouse and talking about the issue, since the well spouse will almost certainly deny the problem. There's no way to clear the air. You might be able to talk to other family members or friends, which might be helpful, but there's little they can do practically to solve the dilemma.

It can helpful to recognize that anger and frustration are merely symptoms; the underlying feelings are usually fear, hurt, or sadness.

Children in this position also tend to spend a lot of time worrying, not just about the parent with dementia but also about the well spouse who may be harming his or her own health and emotional well-being.

Another problem is guilt. Children often feel guilty that they can't help the parent with dementia more, even though their efforts to do so are being blocked. But they can also feel guilty for complaining about the well spouse. After all the well spouse is going to great effort to take care of the other parent and protecting the child from what could otherwise be an enormous burden. In addition most children have a natural feeling of deference to their parents, and it can feel very uncomfortable to challenge a parent's decision about how to take care of a spouse. Some children become martyrs, suppressing their feelings and simply doing whatever the well spouse asks.

In many families, this situation brings out whatever underlying emotional issues the child may have with the well parent or stepparent. Resentments or problems that have been buried for many years can suddenly resurface in the crucible of taking care of someone with dementia.

The Ideal Solution

There's not really an "ideal" solution to this problem, but the best outcome under the circumstances is usually to develop a new relationship with your well parent. Here's a way that the problem is *sometimes* solved, although this solution doesn't always work and it requires a great deal of care.

Denial is a system, like a circuit. Parents who are in denial behave in a way that causes their children to behave in a way that permits the denial to continue. Usually the key is that the well parent exploits the child's natural deference as well as genuine concern for the parent with dementia.

Typically the well parent can suppress any discussion of the other parent's condition by simply denying it. If the child disagrees, the parent can make the child feel disobedient and guilty and can also play the trump card that the parent knows better because he or she lives with the suffering parent and has more information. When the situation gets out of hand and the well parent needs the child's help, the well parent assumes that the child will do whatever is necessary out of love for the other parent.

The problem is that this is untenable for the child. The child is denied important medical information and as a result can't have a straightforward and honest relationship with either parent. The child can't do important planning that would make life much easier down the road. Even worse, when a crisis occurs, the child is expected to drop everything and do whatever is necessary, sacrificing work and family obligations. Even when a crisis doesn't occur, knowing that one could occur at any time means that the child has to live permanently on call, which disrupts work and family and emotional equilibrium.

In order to remedy this, a good goal is to change the family dynamic by getting the well parent to see through the denial and face reality. At the deepest level, the well parent is refusing to accept the eventuality of the spouse's death and the grief that accompanies it. Enabling the well parent to accept that the spouse has a terminal illness—which might involve an intervention by a counselor, social worker, or therapist—is usually the breakthrough that reorients a family toward more appropriate ways of handling the disease.

Obtaining a spouse's acceptance can be incredibly difficult. Acceptance is often described as the last stage of grief. Many well spouses aren't ready for it and won't be for some time. This is especially true if the spouse with dementia is otherwise physically healthy and retains some communication skills and social graces well into the disease process, because it's easier to deny the reality of the impending loss.

Many well spouses find the idea of even the most general discussion of death to be extremely uncomfortable because they imagine that it means "giving up" on the other spouse (which is certainly not true).

Often the first step in changing the family dynamic is for the child to refuse to accept the "on call" arrangement as untenable and instead tell the parent what help is possible and what is too much to ask. If that means that the well parent must allow outside caretaking help or make use of a care facility, then that is the reality. The child is not being mean to draw these lines but rather is simply acknowledging the facts of the disease. A child who has other work and family obligations cannot simply sacrifice them because a parent won't face the truth.

Although it can be hard for adult children to set limits and boundaries in this way, some accomplish it by visualizing what they will tell their own children years from now. They may ask themselves, "Do I want to tell my children that I simply put my family's entire life on hold for 5 years so that my parent could continue pretending to be able to handle something?"

Ideally providing a reality check in the form of being realistic about what you can and cannot do is a way to prompt parents to give in and become more realistic about what they can and cannot do. It's important to note that a reality check is not an ultimatum. In fact very often it takes quite a few conversations to make your point. It's best to be prepared for this possibility. It's also important to note that it's what you do, not what you say you'll do, that will have the greatest effect, because if you draw a boundary and then ignore it in practice, your parent won't take it seriously in the future.

Some other types of conversations can help in this process. One is to keep bringing the subject back to the goals of care. Parents who are focused on their own role in the caregiving process can sometimes be redirected by asking them to describe their own baseline expectations, such as how often the spouse should be bathed or how long the spouse should go before having a wet diaper changed. As a more general matter, parents will often agree on the general goals of the spouse's safety and quality of life. The conversation can then be directed to the best way to accomplish the parent's own stated goals.

Another conversation worth having is about the parent's desire to protect the child. You can gently point out that your parent's behavior is not in fact protecting you; it's depriving you of the ability to organize your own life as well as the satisfaction of participating in your other parent's care.

Yet another conversation could be about what it means to be a care provider. Many well parents believe that if they bring in outside help or put their spouse in a care facility, they will no longer be the spouse's primary care provider. You can explain to your parent that this is incorrect and that just because spouses aren't always providing day-to-day hands-on help doesn't mean that they're not still the primary caregiver and decision maker.

It's often helpful for children to speak with a therapist or other counselor who can help them with their own feelings and provide insight into what the well spouse is going through.

When a breakthrough occurs and honest communication about the previously taboo subject of the disease and death becomes possible, many families find that their entire relationship improves. They become able to make the most of the parent with dementia's later years, and they emerge from the experience stronger and closer and not just exhausted and burned out.

But it's important to note that this "ideal" solution doesn't always work. You have to be cautious in deciding whether it's worth trying. *The most important goal is the safety and health of your parent with dementia*, and you don't want to do anything that will imperil that.

Other Solutions

Short of changing the family dynamic, there are some steps that you may be able to take to make the situation better.

Talk to a therapist. You're going through a lot of emotional difficulty. Talking to a professional can help you process your feelings and come up with helpful coping strategies.

Go to a family dementia support group. You'll meet other people who are going through the same experience and can share what's worked for them.

Involve a social worker, care manager, or other professional. If your well parent will allow it, a professional can often be invaluable in providing perspective.

Talk to the doctor who is caring for your parent with dementia. If you don't think your well parent is being completely honest with you, your other parent's doctor might be. Of course doctors might be limited in what they can tell you because of medical privacy laws. But remember that medical privacy laws limit what a doctor can tell you; they don't limit what you can tell a doctor. Sharing your concerns about the situation can help the doctor to better understand what's going on with the well parent and possibly address treatment accordingly. Keep in mind that doctors who have had experience with dementia are often familiar with the problem of denial and appreciate getting input from other family members who have different perspectives.

Don't argue with your well parent. It's impossible to argue someone out of denial because denial isn't based on logic; it's based on fear. Confronting well parents and saying that they're trying to do too much—or worse, not providing appropriate care—is likely only to provoke a defensive response. This type of confrontation can be tempting but it serves no purpose. It's more helpful to recognize that the root cause is fear, and whenever possible sympathize with the fear and anxiety that your well parent must be experiencing.

If the problem is that your well parent won't let you help at all, there might be ways to offer help that don't trigger the parent's sense of failure. For instance, some children offer help while pretending that the parent with dementia is simply experiencing normal aging. Some tell their well parent how much satisfaction it gives them to take care of the parent with dementia, so the well parent feels that allowing the child to help is a form of caretaking in itself. Some ask the well parent to "teach" them how to take care of the other parent and let them practice doing so "in case it ever becomes necessary." Some manage to persuade their well parent that both parents should move into assisted living together, so the parent with dementia can get specialized treatment if necessary but the well parent can continue providing care.

If you're trying to talk your well parent into allowing outside help or moving the other parent into a care facility, it can be helpful to be honest about how awful this feels and to say how bad you feel about it yourself. Many people experience dread, especially about moving someone into a care facility, because the family knows what's happening and the loved one doesn't. If you can acknowledge the dread and affirmatively make a plan for coping with the feeling, it can be much more effective than simply emphasizing how much the move is necessary and ignoring how heart wrenching it is.

Develop an emergency plan. Know what will happen in a crisis. Will your parent with dementia live with you or with another sibling? If a care facility becomes necessary in a hurry, have you found one or more that you like in advance? Knowing what will happen if something goes very wrong is an important practical step and will also give you some peace of mind.

A Very Different Problem

Sometimes a well spouse will take care of the spouse with dementia for a long time and eventually move the person into a care facility. Then, while the person is still alive, the well spouse will begin dating or become romantically involved with someone else.

Children can have very different reactions to this event. Some children are happy that their parents or stepparents have found a new person in their life who can support them emotionally. But others are very upset and feel that the well spouse is cheating on the still-living parent. This is a difficult conundrum that can have moral as well as psychological dimensions.

One way of looking at the situation is that a well spouse who has spent years taking care of a partner may be at a different stage of the grieving process than a child who hasn't been involved to the same degree in the partner's day-to-day care. The well spouse may have accepted that the partner is no longer there in the same way and have fully grieved the loss. The child might not be in the same emotional place and feel very differently about the matter.

Another issue is that parents and children simply have different relationships. You will only ever have one mother and father, and they are irreplaceable. But it's not unnatural for people who lose a romantic partner—even a very long-term romantic partner—to find another. A child and a spouse may both love the same person intensely, but they will nevertheless see the person in different ways.

Once again there's no easy solution, but talking through your feelings can be very helpful.

10

Taking Care of Yourself Is Not an Afterthought

There are a number of books written by doctors that instruct family members about how to take care of someone with dementia. Often they contain a brief chapter with a title like "Don't Forget to Take Care of Yourself." The typical advice is to remember to eat well, exercise, and get enough sleep. This is of course good (if simplistic) advice. The problem is that these books never explain how you're supposed to find the time to do these things when your world has been turned upside down by your parent's disease.

The answer might seem counterintuitive, but it's true: You have to make taking care of yourself every bit as important as taking care of your parent. (That's why Chapter 8 suggests "respecting your own boundaries" as a goal of your new relationship.)

Part of the reason that this idea seems counterintuitive can be found in thinking about the term *caregiver*, which is often applied to someone caring for a parent with dementia. The word suggests that providing care for someone else is the *job*—it's the main thing you do, your chief responsibility. And if that's your job, then taking care of yourself must be something else—perhaps a leisure-time activity, something you can fit in if you occasionally find that you have the time. And the obvious problem is that, if you're caring for someone with dementia, it's very unlikely that you'll find you have the time.

The fundamental flaw in this approach to caregiving is that it simply doesn't work. You don't become a better caregiver by caring for the other person first and treating your own needs as an afterthought. You become a better caregiver by taking care of your own needs first, and doing so well enough that you have the ability to be energetic, creative, and thoughtful about taking care of someone else.

This approach has been shown to work scientifically. For instance, a study at the University of California at Berkeley followed a large group of people with dementia and their families and measured how much stress the family care providers were under and their general mental health. The study found that on average *people with dementia lived more than a year longer* if their family members were mentally healthy and didn't let themselves become excessively stressed, anxious, or depressed as a result of their responsibilities.

Why? The authors of the study believed that family members who are stressed and don't take care of themselves may overlook important elements of care for dementia sufferers, have more trouble perceiving their needs, or indirectly influence them to react to situations emotionally in a negative way, which can affect their immune system or otherwise cause their own health to become worse.

Although the authors didn't mention it, a common problem is that family members who don't take care of themselves can start to feel resentment toward their loved ones with dementia. And that resentment can be subtly communicated to the loved ones, making them feel ashamed and less likely to try to communicate their needs and ask for help.

And of course family members who don't take care of themselves may become sick and therefore be unable to look after the person with dementia.

By the way, this is one reason why the term "caregiver" is used less and less to describe family members of dementia sufferers. A popular new term is "care partner," which emphasizes that family members are not just unpaid and overworked personal-care aides but rather equal partners of their loved ones with dementia who have their own needs that must be respected. You're a partner, not an employee.

Some people will object to this advice and say that putting your own needs first is selfish. But it's important to remember that there's a difference between interests and needs. Truly self-centered people might put their own interests ahead of those of their parents, with the result that the parents are neglected and uncared for. That really would be selfish. But "needs" are things that you, well, *need* in order to function yourself and in turn to care for someone else. If you neglect your own needs, the person you're caring for will suffer too. Making caring for yourself a priority first is *not* selfish—it's the secret of being able to care for someone else effectively and to keep that person healthy as well.

Put Your Own Mask on First

You've probably heard the familiar airplane safety instructions at the start of each flight. During the part about oxygen masks, after explaining how to use and adjust the masks, the instructions always say, "Be sure to put on your own mask before helping others."

Why? Because if you're getting enough oxygen yourself, you're better able to help a child or an elderly person. If you try to help the other person first—especially if the other person is confused or upset—you might pass out before you succeed. There's a risk that you'll both run out of air.

Caring for someone with dementia is exactly the same: If you're not taking care of yourself first, you're less able to care for someone else.

To take another example, did you know that a large part of lifeguard training is not about how to rescue a drowning person, but about how lifeguards can avoid being drowned themselves during a rescue? That's because people who get into trouble in the water and start to panic will instinctively grab onto anything nearby—including a lifeguard—and push them down into the water in an effort to pull themselves up. Lifeguards spend a lot of time being trained in how not to drown in this way. People who attempt to rescue a drowning person without such training are at risk of dying themselves—so much so in fact that there's a name for the phenomenon: AVIR syndrome, for "aquatic victim instead of rescuer."

In much the same way, people with dementia inadvertently make tremendous demands on their care partners. It's not their fault; they may be panicked by what is happening to them or simply need a lot of attention. But care partners who don't discipline themselves can sometimes end up with "dementia victim instead of rescuer" syndrome.

Some family members use the metaphor of a gas tank. If they don't occasionally stop and refill their tank by attending to their own needs, the car will stop and no one will be able to get where they need to go. (This is another reason the term *care partner* is better than *caregiver*— you can't just give all the time if your tank becomes empty.)

A Healthy Relationship

One of the reasons this book talks about you and your parent having "a new relationship" is that it's good to think of it as a relationship. If you think of yourself simply as a caregiver, you don't have a relationship; you have a *role*—and it can be hard to step out of that role to take care of yourself.

In a healthy relationship, two people each have their own lives. They do what is necessary to take care of themselves, and as a result when they're together, they can bring their full healthy selves to the other person. Of course when parents have dementia, they can't bring a full healthy self to the relationship. But it's far better if at least one person is trying to bring a healthy self than if neither person is.

In our society, a lot of people assume the role of a caregiver professionally—doctors, nurses, social workers, physical therapists, home health aides, and so on. But there's a crucial difference, which is that for these people, caregiving really is a *job*. They get paid, they get benefits, they have work-related interactions, and they receive a certain recognition and status as a result of what they do. What's more, they can leave work and go home and forget about it. There's a point at which their responsibilities simply end.

Despite all this, many health care professionals have trouble leaving work behind. Many of them receive extensive training in setting and enforcing boundaries so that their own mental health and well-being aren't negatively affected by their work.

Of course, as a family member, you can't simply treat what you do as a job. You don't get a salary, you don't have a title, and you can't simply "clock out" at the end of the day. What you have is a relationship. So the best approach is to treat it as a real relationship, respect your own boundaries, and put your own needs first so you can stay mentally and physically healthy enough to provide your parent with the best care you can.

What's the Secret?

Putting your own needs first is certainly easier said than done. But just resolving to do it is a big step in the right direction.

It's also worth recognizing why most people *don't* put their own needs first. The reason is that very few people step back and actually think about their own needs. Dementia caregivers have a tendency to think about their needs only when something they particularly need has been lacking for so long that they experience intense frustration or a catastrophic problem. And of course by that time it's too late.

So it's a good idea to ponder your own needs and how you can meet them. Writing them down is a good idea. Simply articulating what you need is a crucial first step in making sure that you take care of yourself.

It's about Time

As noted at the beginning of this chapter, three important needs that are often mentioned in books on caring for people with dementia are eating well, exercising, and getting enough sleep, all of which maintain your physical health. Other needs, such as relaxation, recreation, hobbies, and having a social life, are essential to your mental health.

Having a parent with dementia interferes with these needs not because the disease causes parents to suddenly demand that you stop going to the gym, but because caregiving takes up so much *time*. The one factor that all these needs have in common is that they too take time. When people start taking care of someone with dementia, their free time disappears. In order to cope, they gradually cut these activities out of their life.

At first, of course, not meeting some of your needs is manageable. No one suffers greatly because of skipping exercise occasionally, missing an evening with friends, or staying up late one night. But over time, as people skip important activities more and more regularly, doing so takes its toll. They become tired, irritable, stressed, short-tempered, nervous, and unhealthy. And none of this is good for the person they're taking care of.

So the first step in meeting these needs is to figure out how much time you need for yourself. This may seem like an odd exercise, but it's important. How much sleep do you need each night to feel okay? How often do you need to exercise? How much time per month do you need to devote to hobbies, getting together with friends, and so on in order not to be impaired by stress?

Of course whatever number you come up with might prove to be impossible to achieve in practice. But at least you have a goal.

It's also a good idea to actually schedule leisure activities, because then you will feel some responsibility to take care of yourself instead of having your self-care always be an afterthought that can be preempted by something else. Planning ahead to read a good book for an hour on Tuesday night might seem very odd, but that's because this kind of conscious self-care wasn't necessary before your parent had dementia.

Making the Time

Manufacturing free time might seem impossible, but it becomes easier if you schedule your relaxation. It forces you to find ways to make room for it.

A next step is to ask for help. You might have relatives or family friends who are willing to provide assistance. If they are, make a list of things they can do. Be specific: Can they shop for you on Wednesday? Can they do a cleaning project? Can they sit with your parent for an hour or two on Sunday? Many people appreciate general offers of help but are unwilling to ask for specific favors. Don't be. You need to make time for yourself so you can better care for your parent.

Keep in mind too that most people don't understand what a person with dementia needs and, while they might be willing to help, they have no idea what would actually be useful to you. They might very much appreciate being given a specific project (or a few options of specific projects).

Many people are surprised to find out who is willing to help and who isn't. They might be resentful because family members who are "supposed" to be willing to help aren't, whereas a neighbor who has no obligation is willing to play cards with your parent for hours on the weekends. In general it's not a good idea to waste time trying to shame people into helping you if they're unwilling. Accept help where you can get it.

It's also good to practice discerning how much of your time your parent actually needs as opposed to how much of your time he or she wants. A parent's wants may be unlimited! But remember that you're asking what's most important at this moment, you're focusing on a "good enough" relationship, and you're respecting your own boundaries.

Parents with dementia often insist that they "need" you to do something for them, when in fact they're just scared or confused and they want reassurance and comfort. Very often, if you listen to what they are feeling (and not just their words) and you provide them with sympathy and reassurance, their "need" will magically go away.

Dementia caregivers also have a tendency to multiply their parents' needs. As they gradually take over more and more aspects of their parents' lives, they want to handle things in the way that seems best to them. The result unfortunately can be "mission creep." Instead of just paying bills, they end up cleaning out the garage or taking on other helpful-but-not-strictly-necessary household tasks. It's always good to reflect on whether a task you're doing for your parent is truly necessary, and if it's not whether it's worth your time.

Another way to create more free time is to use grocery-delivery and other errand services. These services may cost more and you'll lose some control over how tasks are done, but the added expense may be worth it to create time for yourself.

A further option is to hire aides for a few hours a week to help with personal care, to use group day care services for people with dementia, or to hire an occasional companion. These options involve more expense—and your parent may object at first—but they can all give you time to restore your sanity.

Some dementia-care facilities offer respite care, where your parent can stay for a short period of time without being a permanent resident. This can be a very good option if you need to take a vacation. Even if the other options can buy you a few hours here and there, sometimes there is no psychological substitute for a sustained period of getting away from pressing responsibilities.

Relieving Stress

Another type of need you'll undoubtedly have is relieving stress. Of course exercising, sleeping enough, relaxation, and talking with friends are all good ways of relieving stress. But the unique demands of caring for someone with dementia may leave you with more stress than you can easily handle.

For this reason, it can be good to engage in practices that are specifically designed to reduce stress. For instance meditation and yoga have both been shown to help people stay calm in extremely difficult situations.

It's also a good idea to be aware of your own stress level and reflect on exactly what causes the stress. In general stress is caused by a desire to control a situation that you can't truly control. The gap between what you want to happen and what you can actually make happen is what causes the stress. If you feel stressed, it's useful to reflect on the fact that, try as you might and however much you want to, you can't actually control your parent's situation.

It's hard to accept this fact, but you can't cure dementia, you can't provide perfect care, and you can't change other people's personalities. All you can do is be yourself.

Dementia is painful, and your parent will suffer and experience a lot of unhappiness; that's simply the nature of the disease. We of course want to "fix" the pain, but there's a limit to what we can do. Often we can't fix anything; all we can do is be present and sympathetic.

But because that's all we can do, that's enough. The goal is to have a good enough relationship. If we can't fix it, we can sympathize. This is a sad reality, but accepting it allows us to let go of the stress and focus on being present to the situation.

Coping with Loss

A final need that dementia caregivers have is coping with the loss and emotional sadness that come with the disease.

Some people see a therapist to talk about what they're experiencing, and therapy can be very helpful in working through their feelings.

An additional option is to join one of the many dementia caregiver support groups that have sprung up lately. Talking with and getting to know other people who are dealing with a parent with dementia can be enormously useful for a number of reasons.

For one thing, dementia robs parents of their ability to provide emotional support to their adult children, who often don't get much support from their other family members and friends because they simply don't understand the pressure and difficulty that children face. Unless you've been there, it's very difficult to comprehend. For another, the kinds of grief that care partners feel is not well understood in society. Family members grieve a loss, but it's not the same as a death that other people can understand. However, fellow dementia caregivers often have a good sense of all the emotions you're going through. In addition support groups can provide you with helpful tips and caregiving strategies, connections to local resources, and what is in effect an expanded social life.

III

Caring Smarter, Not Harder

11

What It Means to Care Smarter

As mentioned in the introduction, you may have heard the expression *Work smarter, not harder*. The title of this part of the book is "Care Smarter, Not Harder." That's because caring for someone with dementia is not about exhausting yourself in an impossible effort to do everything, but identifying the most important tasks and doing them as effectively as possible.

After you've established goals for your new relationship, the next step is developing the skills to put them into practice. Most people never think of caring for someone with dementia as a skill or as involving a series of skills. At the outset, providing care for a dementia sufferer doesn't seem to involve any particular skills, just handling tasks that another person can no longer handle alone.

And yet nothing could be further from the truth. As the disease progresses, interacting with a parent becomes more and more difficult and requires carefully using certain techniques to get an optimal result. They are not difficult skills to acquire, and they don't involve a lot of time or specialized education or medical training. Anyone can learn them and develop them with some practice. But most people never do—which is why they so often end up expending enormous amounts of energy and effort and getting minimal or negative results. They work harder and harder, when they should be working smarter.

These skills are almost never taught by doctors or other medical professionals. Most people learn them, if at all, through lengthy trial and error. But if you can start thinking about them as early as possible, you can make your role of caring for your parent far easier than it otherwise would be.

Each skill corresponds to a unique type of behavioral challenge posed by the disease, and they are all discussed in the following chapters. Among others, they include the following:

- How to communicate with your parent

- How to avoid problems with your parent's finances

- How to keep your parent safe at home

- How to get outside help

- How to deal with a parent who can no longer drive safely

- How to handle problem behaviors—those that are disruptive, dangerous, or embarrassing

- How to manage moving a parent to a care facility if it becomes necessary

These skills all have the immediate benefit of making your life easier and reducing the stress of caring for a parent with dementia. But they can also help you to achieve the most important goal of all, which is making your new relationship as close and rewarding as it can be under the circumstances.

12

How to Communicate
with a Parent with Dementia

I n most cases, the core problem in dealing with a parent with dementia is the inability to communicate. It's hard enough when parents can't do things for themselves or can't be trusted to manage on their own safely. But this difficulty is magnified many times over when parents can't express what they're thinking and feeling . . . and you can't explain to them what you're doing, what you need for them to do, and what your reasons are.

In the early stages of dementia, this problem is usually not so bad. Parents may forget something but they can carry on once they're reminded of it. Parents may have trouble finding words, but they can generally find a way to make themselves understood.

As the disease progresses, however, the problem gets worse. You can usually carry on a conversation with someone whose sentences are occasionally missing a word or contain the wrong word. But when a sentence is missing half its words, it becomes far more difficult.

That's not to say that it's impossible to communicate with someone with moderate dementia. However, you can't communicate in the way that you normally do. Effective communication (or as-effective-as-possible communication) requires in effect learning a new language, or at least learning to use language in a very different way.

Using language in this new way is a skill. With some practice, it's a skill you can definitely master. The funny thing about this skill is that it's seldom obvious that you've acquired it. It's not like becoming very good at playing the piano, which means you can perform something that clearly demonstrates your accomplishment to everyone. Other people might not even realize that you're using this skill at all. But what they *will* notice is that you consistently have much more effective interactions with your parent than they do.

The Middle of a Novel

An important key to learning this new skill is to think about the world from your parent's perspective.

It's hard to imagine what the world is like for someone with dementia, but here's an exercise that can help. If you own a novel that you haven't read, open it to a random page in the middle and read just that page. What do you find? You can probably get a very vague understanding of the action, a sense of the mood, and perhaps some idea about a character or two. You can probably tell if you're meant to experience drama, suspense, humor, or some other emotion. But you don't really know what's going on. You can't understand what is happening and why because you haven't read the previous chapters. You have no *memory*. And because you have no memory, you have no ability to put the page you've just read into context.

Your parent is going through a similar experience. He or she might have a general sense of who people are and what they're doing in the present moment. But what your parent lacks is the ability to put experience into context and therefore to make sense of what is happening.

Therefore one of the keys to effective communication is to continually supply context for your parent.

This is actually something that we do naturally in certain other situations. For instance, imagine that you have a group of close friends who have known each other for a long time and have a lot of history, stories, and in-jokes. Then a new person joins your group. A certain amount of your time will be spent explaining background information, relationships, and obscure references. You have a sense that the new person has opened your novel in the middle and that you need to explain your backstory so that he or she isn't mystified.

Another example would be doctors and dentists who explain each thing they're about to do during a procedure so that the patient doesn't feel confused, surprised, or upset.

It's hard to realize that you need to provide context for your parent because *it's your parent*. Your parent is *supposed* to know the backstory. But dementia takes this ability away.

How to Provide Context

It's possible to provide context in a subtle way, simply by including information. "Mom," you might say, "this is Helen. She's your aide and she's here to help you take a bath." Saying this is far easier and less confusing for your parent than having someone she might not recognize simply arrive and suddenly begin trying to take her clothes off.

"Dad," you might say, "this is Barbara, who's married to your son Bill." This information helps your father and also spares him the embarrassment of asking who she is. (Later on, you might need to say, "Hi Dad, it's your daughter Susan.")

It's good to get into the habit of explaining anything you do or any change you make to the environment. "I'm turning the television off so that it will be easier for us to talk." "I'm getting you a sweater because it's cold today." "I'm going to the kitchen to get a drink of water and I'll be right back." "We're going to the eye doctor today to see if you need new glasses." Continually supplying context will help your parent to stay calm and oriented. It's one of the most effective forms of communication.

Another good practice when communicating context is to avoid the use of pronouns as much as possible. Pronouns are words such as *he, she, his, her, it,* and so on. They're short words that substitute for longer words because it's assumed that the person we're talking with knows what they refer to. But with dementia sufferers, that's a dangerous assumption. "He'll put it in his car" can be very confusing. "Your son-in-law Jim will put your purse in the car so you'll have it while we're riding" supplies far more context.

When people use a lot of pronouns, parents with dementia sometimes feel like everyone around them is speaking in code. They may become paranoid and think that people are talking behind their back or otherwise trying to keep them from knowing what's going on. Avoiding pronouns is a good way to keep your parent from thinking this way.

Of course it can sound stilted to talk without pronouns. (And eliminating them altogether is impossible.) Nevertheless being aware of your use of pronouns and minimizing them as much as you can is often very helpful.

Occasionally a parent might snap at you for using these context-providing techniques. "I know who Barbara is!" he might say angrily. "You don't have to talk down to me like that!" Of course the truth is that he might or might not have known who Barbara was if you didn't tell him. It's easy to become defensive when you're snapped at like this, but it's important to remember that the comment is not about you. Your parent is simply frustrated with himself because he needs to have the context explained and is expressing that frustration in the only way that he can think of at the moment. You can simply ignore the comment and continue subtly providing contextual information.

Avoiding Agitation

Difficulty in communication is a key reason dementia sufferers become agitated—it's frustrating not to be able to make yourself understood or to understand others. So, it's a good idea to try to communicate in a way that reduces the likelihood of agitation.

One way to do this is to speak in a calm, measured, even tone. This can be difficult to do, especially if you're in a hurry, but it's worth putting in the effort. It's a bit like acting—you're adopting the persona of a person who is relaxed, calm, and soothing. The reason is that, since your parent has difficulty understanding the context of situations, he or she will look to your manner to obtain clues as to how to feel and respond. If you seem nervous, your parent will likely feel nervous too. If you seem happy and relaxed, your parent will get the subtle message that there's nothing to be worried about. It can be difficult to remain calm if your parent is agitated—or even saying things that hurt or upset you—but staying relentlessly calm is the quickest way to defuse the situation.

It can also be good to try to lower the pitch of your voice. Lower-pitched voices are generally perceived as calmer (and in addition they can be easier to understand for people who have mild hearing loss).

Some people approach communicating with dementia sufferers by talking to them in a singsong way, as though they were little children. Occasionally using a singsong voice does make people with dementia seem happy. However, if they become worried or agitated, a singsong manner can make the problem worse by causing them to feel as though they are being infantilized and not taken seriously. In general a calm, measured tone works better because it communicates dignity and respect.

Speaking of dignity and respect, some parents with dementia become irritated when their family members repeatedly supply missing words for them. Most of the time doing so is helpful, but sometimes parents would prefer to be given extra time to remember the word on their own. Being sensitive to your parent's preferences—or even asking in a lucid moment which they prefer—shows respect and can have a calming effect.

Some other tips include:

- Begin by saying the person's name (or "Mom" or "Dad"), which gives the person time to focus on listening to you.

- Maintain eye contact when speaking.

- If possible, be at the same eye level, so you're sitting if your parent is sitting, for example.

- Approach your parent from the front, rather than walking up from the back or the side or calling your parent from another room.

- Avoid sudden movements, which can be distracting or worrying.

All of these tips demonstrate respect and can help keep your parent from having the sense of being "managed."

Another technique to avoid agitation is to couch statements as much as possible in a positive way. For instance rather than telling your parent *not* to do something—which can cause defensiveness—you can redirect your parent toward something else.

Instead of telling your mother not to go outside, for example, you might say, "Let's go into the living room." Instead of telling your father not to eat something with his fingers, you might say, "Here, it'll be easier if you use a fork." Instead of "You're in the wrong place," you can smile and say, "It looks like you're looking for the kitchen. Here, it's this way."

Parents with dementia already know that they make a lot of mistakes, and they likely feel unhappy and self-conscious about it. Offering a positive alternative, rather than suggesting that parents did something else "wrong," can go a long way toward keeping them from getting upset.

You can also use this technique if you're tempted to complain about the monotony of your parent's routine. Instead of making a negative comment about doing the same thing over and over, you can say, "Gee, let's try something new!"

Parents will almost always be calmer if they not only are able to understand you, but can also feel that you understand *them*. Thus it can be a very good idea, when a parent expresses something, to summarize back what was said and ask if you understood correctly. This not only makes sure you *did* understand correctly, but also reassures parents that they have been heard.

Another tip is that there's seldom a need to tell a parent in advance about appointments or other upcoming events. Dementia sufferers often retain memories of emotions much longer than memories of facts. As a result, when parents with dementia hear that they have a doctor's appointment tomorrow, it's unlikely that they will be able to remember the details, but they might be left with a gnawing worry that there's something they need to do or something that is expected of them. Such worrying can lead to agitation. It's usually better to simply wait until the appointed time and then say, "We need to go to the doctor for a routine checkup."

Dealing with Cognitive Deficits

Other important techniques that are part of communicating more effectively are based on responding to the primary cognitive deficits caused by dementia. They include loss of memory, loss of language skills, and loss of focus and reasoning ability.

LOSS OF MEMORY

People who are having trouble with their memory will repeat themselves a lot. They'll ask the same question or make the same comment over and over again. They'll also need information to be repeated to them a lot. Just because you told your parent 5 minutes ago about a medical appointment today doesn't mean that you won't need to repeat this information a few more times.

This kind of repetition can be very frustrating to care partners. One of the reasons is that it's like a microcosm of caring for someone with dementia in general: There's a sense that you never make any progress. People have a feeling of satisfaction when they sense that all their work is accomplishing something and making a difference. But when you keep telling parents some piece of information and they simply can't retain it, the result is a feeling of futility—like nothing you do has any value or effect. This can be very disheartening and ultimately frustrating to care partners.

One solution in this situation is to remember the goal of listening to feelings and not just words—as well as responding with feelings and not just words. Because the content of your conversation appears to go "in one ear and out the other," it's good to recognize that the content isn't really very important. The important point is to use the conversation as an occasion to express affection and reassurance. You can make a game of saying the same thing over and over or responding to the same question again and again, but always in a way that expresses emotional closeness. This kind of response will be more valuable for your parent and much more satisfying for you.

Another good strategy for coping with loss of memory is to avoid quizzing your parent. Questions such as, "Where did you put your glasses?" or "Did David come to see you this morning?" are unlikely to be productive or useful. Your parent will probably have forgotten and may well be embarrassed by this fact. Worse, your parent might become defensive, frustrated, or angry about being put on the spot.

In addition even if your parent gives you an answer, there's no reason to think that it will be the correct one. Your mother might tell you that David didn't come to visit because she can't remember the visit, for instance, or might say that David *did* come to visit because David came to visit a few days ago, and she is confused about what day it is. And so on.

Asking questions about what happened to someone recently or what the person has been doing is normally a polite way to start a conversation, but with someone with dementia it's generally a bad idea. And if you truly need information, it's almost always better if possible to find some other way to get an answer.

A final technique for dealing with loss of memory is based on the fact that people with dementia tend to lose their short-term memory before their long-term memory. Often, they can remember something that happened 30 years ago but not something that happened 30 minutes ago. When starting a conversation therefore it's frequently a good idea to reminisce—to talk about pleasant or funny memories that your parent has from many years ago. This approach often leads to much more enjoyable interactions than asking about what has happened since the last time you visited.

LOSS OF LANGUAGE SKILLS

Your parent's loss of language skills can make it difficult for him or her to communicate with you—to find the right words to express ideas. But importantly, this cognitive problem can also make it hard for you to communicate with your parent. Parents often have a great deal of difficulty comprehending and processing what their children are saying to them.

Here's something that might help you to understand your parent's condition: Perhaps you studied a foreign language in school. You might have spent a few years learning basic grammar and vocabulary, but you never lived in a foreign country or became fluent. Imagine that you suddenly found yourself among a group of native speakers and were expected to keep up with their conversation. You might be able to get a general sense of the topic, but you would miss a lot of words and subtleties and feel confused much of the time.

What would help you in this situation? Probably you would want everyone to speak much more slowly, to enunciate clearly, to use simpler vocabulary, and to avoid idioms and figures of speech that are hard for foreigners to grasp.

It's the same with a person with dementia. If you want to be understood, it's good to speak slowly, clearly, and simply.

Many people don't realize how complex their speech normally is. A sentence such as "I'm going to stop at the convenience store on the way home from work and pick up some more paper towels because it looks like we're running low" is easily understood by most people, but it can be very difficult for a person with dementia to process. By contrast "I will buy more paper towels" communicates the same essential facts but in a way that is much easier to follow.

Figures of speech come so naturally to native speakers that much of the time we don't even realize that we're using them, but it's good to try to be aware of them and generally avoid them. Proverbs are one example. Saying "Better safe than sorry" or "Things always happen for a reason" may leave your parent mystified. Idioms are another example. Many people might say, "I'm going to quickly run out to the post office," but a parent with dementia might imagine that you plan to literally run there.

Slang terms—even common slang expressions, such as "what's up?" or "no big deal"—can leave parents scratching their heads.

Jokes can be very difficult for a person with dementia to grasp, unless they are very simple or silly. That's because many jokes require thinking of something in one way and then suddenly thinking of the same thing in a different way, which is a skill that people with dementia lose.

In general any type of language that is not meant to be taken completely literally—including sarcasm and innuendo—is difficult for dementia sufferers. Abstract concepts can also be difficult for them to process. It's usually best to stick to simple, concrete language, and to imagine how you would talk to a nonnative speaker.

Another key to communicating is to use body language, gestures, and inflection. All these nonverbal ways of communicating help a person with dementia to "get" what you're saying, because they provide additional clues to your meaning. It's perfectly okay to slightly exaggerate gestures and inflection in order to help get your message across.

It's extremely common for families of dementia sufferers to find that it's much easier to communicate in person than on the phone. Quite apart from the fact that people with dementia have difficulty using phones and remembering numbers and messages, talking on the phone means that you can't use gestures, facial expressions, and body language to make your point. Without these clues, it can be a lot harder to be understood. (Many people with dementia eventually try to avoid using phones altogether for this reason.)

As video phone services become more common, it will be interesting to see the effects for people with dementia. Little research has been done on this development. It's possible that videoconferencing will make communication by phone easier, although it could also end up being more confusing for people with the disease.

LOSS OF FOCUS AND REASONING ABILITY

A common characteristic of people with dementia is that they lose the ability to stay "on track." If you try to have a conversation with them about a topic, or get them to perform a certain task, they will tend to get distracted, change the subject, or lose their focus. That's because the disease impairs their ability to pay attention and to use logic.

Many family members become frustrated when this happens. They will implore their parent to pay more attention—but of course the problem is not that the parent doesn't *want* to pay attention; it's that he or she isn't able to.

Many care partners will also go to some length to reason with parents or try to get them to understand the logic behind something—why they need to take a bath, get dressed, go to the doctor, not go outside, and the like. Very often these attempts are unsuccessful and lead to frustration on both sides.

In such cases, it's worth asking yourself whether it's truly necessary that your parent understand your reasoning. In many cases, it might not be, as long as you can accomplish your goal by some other means. Many children feel guilty about making parents do something that they are reluctant to do, and try to explain the reason for it because it's a way of making themselves feel less guilty—but if their parents can't follow the logic, it might simply make them more upset.

If it *is* necessary for your parent to understand your reasoning, you might find that it's better to wait for another opportunity. Many people with dementia have better skills on some days than on others or at certain times of the day as opposed to at other times.

Because people with dementia so commonly experience distraction, it can be helpful to eliminate any unnecessary noise while you're talking with your parent. For instance you might want to turn off a TV or music in the background.

As with memory loss, the lack of focus and reasoning ability often comes into play when you ask your parent a question, so it's wise to be careful about how you ask questions. For one thing, it often takes people with dementia a long time to process a question and come up with an answer, so you might need to be patient and perhaps repeat the question a few times before you get the response you need.

Open-ended questions—those that don't suggest a particular response—can be especially difficult for dementia sufferers. For instance a question such as "Are you feeling happy today?" is fairly easy to answer, but a more open-ended question such as "How are you feeling today?" can be much more difficult. Parents may be unable to come up with a response and become frustrated at their inability.

"Why" questions are especially difficult to answer because they typically require remembering what happened, remembering what led up to what happened, understanding the connection, and then articulating it. For dementia sufferers, the mental effort needed can sometimes be impossible.

Another tricky type of question is one that offers choices. A question such as "What would you like to do now?" may well be met with a blank look, whereas a more specific question such as "Would you like to go and sit on the patio?" is much easier to answer. Many dementia sufferers can handle a question that offers two choices ("Would you like to sit in the shade or in the sun?" "Would you like the red sweater or the blue one?"), but a question with three or more choices can be much harder to process.

Hearing Aids

Many older people who have dementia also suffer from hearing loss. The hearing problem can obviously compound the person's communication difficulties. Also as people lose their cognitive abilities, they often rely more and more on their senses, such as hearing and vision, to understand what's going on. As a result, hearing loss can make things doubly difficult.

Hearing aid technology has improved considerably in recent years, and while hearing aids are not inexpensive and are still far from perfect, they can help a lot of people to hear better. The problem is that they can be difficult for people with dementia to use. For instance, many people with dementia have difficulty figuring out how to insert them into their ears.

Some hearing aids require frequent battery replacements. Some need to be recharged at night, and some need to be switched on after being recharged. These tasks can be hard for people with dementia to remember to do. The problem is that if you *don't* do them, having hearing aids can actually be worse than not having them. A hearing aid that has lost its charge, has a dead battery, or hasn't been switched on simply plugs up the person's ear canal and makes it harder to hear, not easier.

Hearing aids can also be easy to lose—especially for people who are living in a facility where there are a lot of other people and activities. And some parents with dementia have been known to accidentally throw them away.

There's no perfect solution to this problem. Some older people are very good about letting family members insert and remove their hearing aids. But other families have found that on balance hearing aids are more trouble than they're worth.

13

Avoiding Headaches
with Your Parent's Finances

Frequently one of the first signs that people are developing dementia is that they have trouble handling financial matters. They may have difficulty in balancing a checkbook or otherwise reconciling accounts, monitoring investments, paying bills on time, preparing tax returns, and generally using good financial judgment. They might also become more susceptible to scams and exploitation.

As soon as you suspect that your parent has dementia, one of the most important tasks to take care of is to quickly get a handle on the person's finances. It's essential that arrangements be made so that you (or another relative or trusted person) can manage your parent's affairs once your parent is no longer competent to do so. These arrangements should ideally be made *before* your parent loses the ability to make and understand financial and legal decisions. If you wait until your parent is no longer competent, it may be far more difficult to do what needs to be done. Many families lose a lot of money and experience significant legal headaches because it becomes difficult or impossible to make necessary financial changes after relatives develop dementia and can no longer do so on their own.

There have been cases where people with dementia needed to withdraw money from a bank or investment account in order to pay for care but they could no longer do so themselves, and no one else was authorized to make a withdrawal; cases where investments became wildly inappropriate, but no one was able to make changes to the way the investments were set up; cases where people with dementia could no longer make a will, with the result that their assets didn't go where they would have preferred after death; cases where even though a parent moved out of a house, it was extremely difficult for the children to legally sell it; and cases where bank accounts that no one in the family could access were declared "inactive," and the money was forfeited to the government. And so on.

That's not to say that all is lost if your parent is already incompetent to make financial choices. It's just likely to be more difficult. So as with so many other aspects of dementia, it can pay big dividends to be proactive.

This chapter gives you a general overview of the kinds of issues you need to be aware of. It describes the laws in the United States; the laws may be somewhat different in other countries, although the general outline is likely to be similar. However, wherever you live, it's a good idea to speak to an attorney or trusted financial advisor who is familiar with issues involving senior citizens and in particular those who have dementia. A trained counselor also can explain how the rules apply to your specific situation and give you advice tailored to your exact needs.

Keep in mind that you don't have to be the person who takes over your parent's finances if you don't feel comfortable in that role. The person who handles the day-to-day issues could be another relative or even a professional. But the key is to get a plan in place as early as possible, even if you're not the person who manages all the details going forward.

Avoiding Guardianship

In general the overarching goal in dealing with your parent's finances is to avoid a process called "guardianship." Guardianship (also known as "conservatorship" in some states) is a kind of worst-case scenario for situations in which people can't manage their finances and no one else has been given the authority to do so. In such cases, a court can step in and appoint someone (a family member or sometimes an attorney or other representative) to make financial, legal, and medical decisions on the person's behalf.

This option sounds like a solution, and it is, but it's usually a very bad solution. In order for you or another relative to be appointed as a guardian, you'll have to file a court petition. You'll likely have to hire a lawyer for the purpose and have doctors officially certify that your parent is incapacitated. Filing a court petition and hiring a lawyer can cost a lot of money. The process of getting named as a guardian can drag on for months, during which time no one will be able make any decisions for your parent's benefit. Even after you're named as a guardian, you might still be required to return to court to get a judge's permission for major decisions, such as transferring investments or selling a house. You'll have to keep meticulous records of every expense and file periodic reports with the court regarding nearly every single decision you've made on your parent's behalf. It's expensive, time-consuming, and a nuisance.

As a result, the most important goal is usually to make sure that guardianship is unnecessary by enabling someone to make legal decisions for your parent without having to resort to it. There are other goals too of course, but this one is typically the most critical.

Three Documents

There are three types of documents that almost everyone should have in place to protect themselves in case something unfortunate happens to them, but it's especially critical to have them for someone who is developing dementia. Among other benefits, these documents can help you avoid the necessity of guardianship. You and your parent can work with a lawyer to arrange for the documents to be completed.

1. POWER OF ATTORNEY

A *power of attorney* document authorizes another person to make legal and financial decisions for the person who signs it. This other person is called an *attorney-in-fact*. Having your parent sign a power of attorney allowing you or another relative to make decisions is enormously helpful. It won't solve every problem, but it will make handling these matters a lot easier.

A *durable* power of attorney allows the attorney-in-fact to make decisions for the person as soon as the document is signed. (There's a similar type of document called a *general* power of attorney but, unlike a durable power of attorney, it ceases to be effective if the person becomes incapacitated—so it isn't helpful in the case of dementia.)

A power of attorney document typically spells out all the kinds of decisions that the attorney-in-fact can make. One power you might want to give some thought to is the power to make gifts of the signer's assets. Some power of attorney documents include this as a power that the attorney-in-fact has, but others don't. If the power is not included, it's usually because of a fear that the attorney-in-fact might abuse it. However, your parent might want you or another relative to have the ability to make gifts—especially because doing so in certain situations can have tax advantages.

Another type of document is called a *springing* power of attorney. Unlike a standard durable power of attorney, a springing power of attorney doesn't go into effect as soon as it's signed; it goes into effect only if the signer becomes incapacitated and can't make decisions on his or her own. Many people are more comfortable signing a springing power of attorney because they're not immediately giving someone else full power over their affairs—the power only "springs" into effect if and when it's needed.

There's a downside to springing powers, however. Suppose you walk into a bank and want to withdraw funds from your parent's account in order to pay bills. With a springing power, you can't just show the bank the document; you will also have to prove that your parent is in fact incapacitated. Perhaps the bank will accept a signed letter from your parent's doctor, but it might not; some institutions are very picky. With a durable power of attorney, there are fewer hurdles to overcome.

Springing powers are especially tricky in the case of dementia. When people have a stroke or are in a coma, it might be immediately obvious to everyone that they are incapacitated. But dementia can be much more ambiguous. Many people in the early stages of dementia are competent in certain ways but not in others, or on certain days but not on others, or even at certain times of the day but not at others. A determination that a person with dementia is incompetent might not be simple or clear-cut.

Some institutions are skeptical of power of attorney documents in general. Many financial organizations have their own specific power of attorney forms. If possible, it's a good idea to ask any institution that your parent deals with regularly if it has its own power of attorney form and have your parent fill that out as well. With Medicare and Social Security in particular it's helpful to fill out the applicable government forms.

Some power of attorney documents allow for multiple attorneys-in-fact. For instance, two siblings might both be authorized to make decisions. Many parents like this idea because it means that they don't have to appear to favor one sibling over the other when completing the document. Having two attorneys-in-fact can be useful in some situations, such as if one sibling is unavailable in an emergency.

But there can also be downsides. For instance, the document will need to specify if each attorney-in-fact can act independently or if both must agree on all decisions. If you say that both must agree, then you've added a layer of complexity and paperwork, slowed down decision making, and eliminated the advantage that one person can act in an emergency. On the other hand, if both attorneys-in-fact can act independently, then they might inadvertently act at cross-purposes on occasion. Also many institutions are skeptical about complying with such a document since they fear that if they do what one person says, they might get sued if the other person doesn't approve.

A better alternative may be to name an "alternate" attorney-in-fact who can take over if the main attorney-in-fact resigns or becomes incapacitated. This can be very important if two parents sign power of attorney documents naming each other as the attorney-in-fact. If one parent develops dementia and then the other dies or becomes incapacitated, having an alternate named in the document can be tremendously valuable.

2. HEALTH CARE PROXY AND LIVING WILL

These documents have different names in different states, but whatever they're called, a health care proxy appoints someone else to make medical decisions if the signer can't make them, and a living will (or advance directive) specifies what sorts of medical treatment people want or don't want in certain situations where they can't make their wishes known.

A health care proxy is essentially a power of attorney that covers medical decisions, rather than legal and financial decisions.

Hospitals and other facilities will generally accept decisions made by an incapacitated person's next of kin. If the person is married, the spouse is almost always considered the next of kin. However, it can get more complicated. If the person is widowed or divorced, and has two children, which child is authorized to decide? Does a child take precedence over a spouse who is separated or estranged? A health care proxy can solve these sorts of problems.

A living will typically allows signers to choose what treatments they want or don't want in an emergency as they approach the end of life. For instance, many people specify "do not resuscitate" if they stop breathing or their heart stops beating. Others will say whether they want to be intubated or put on a ventilator.

An increasing number of advance directives offer a "do not transport" or "do not hospitalize" option. These were instituted because a number of very frail elderly people were being repeatedly transferred from nursing homes to hospitals for what seemed like minimal health benefits considering the trauma and disruption that the transfers caused. However, you should be aware that "do not transport" can be a very tricky choice. Lots of older people's lives can easily be saved by going to the hospital, and electing "do not transport" can cause them to die much sooner than they otherwise would.

Because these documents tend to be useful in a crisis, it's worth thinking about where to keep them. A document such as a will can easily be kept in a safe deposit box, for instance, but a health care proxy might not be of much use to you if a decision needs to be made right away and you can't access the document until the bank opens in the morning. The proxy should be kept where you will have easy access to it. And it's a good idea to make sure your parent's doctor has a copy of both the proxy and the living will.

If your parent is serious about the wishes in an advance directive, it should be even more accessible. Some people keep a copy on their refrigerator so that EMTs will be likely to find it.

As with power of attorney documents, it's a good idea for a health care proxy to name an alternate in case the first person named in the proxy is unable to act.

While health care proxies and living wills are important, they're not as critical as powers of attorney when it comes to avoiding guardianship. But they can still be helpful. For instance, if a parent is being kept alive artificially for a long period and family members can't agree on what to do, a court might step in and appoint a guardian to make decisions.

3. WILL AND/OR LIVING TRUST

If your parent doesn't have a will, it's a good idea to see a lawyer and have one drafted before he or she becomes mentally incompetent to sign it. This is also true if your parent wrote a will years ago but it's now outdated. (A will can become outdated if it no longer reflects your parent's preferences, if your parent has gotten divorced, if there are new spouses or grandchildren in the family, or even if the tax laws have been changed since the will was written.)

When parents die without a will or with an outdated will, their assets will probably not be distributed in the ways that they would have wanted. Additionally taxes might become due that could have been avoided. In the United States, the federal estate tax has been limited recently so that it affects only very wealthy individuals, but a number of states have their own estate and inheritance taxes that affect people who are not nearly as wealthy.

Having a will isn't in itself a way to avoid guardianship, but you should know that many older people create *revocable trusts*, sometimes called living trusts, instead of or in addition to writing a will. These trusts own the person's assets and are often used to avoid probate. Typically the person who creates the trust acts as the trustee, but a trust can also have a "disability trustee" who takes over if the person becomes incapacitated—much like a springing power of attorney. You might be able to avoid guardianship proceedings if you can make sure that your parent's living trust has a disability trustee.

In such cases, you'll also want to make sure that the living trust actually owns all your parent's assets. Many people create a living trust to own their financial accounts, for instance, but they never follow through and make sure the accounts are retitled in the trust's name rather than in their individual names. (And this outcome is obviously much more likely if your parent is in the early stages of dementia.)

Make an Inventory

A lot of people are overwhelmed by the idea of managing their parent's finances, but it's often easier than you might think if you start by making a simple inventory of your parent's assets. It might include real estate, bank accounts, investment accounts, retirement accounts such as IRAs and 401(k) plans, and annuities. It might also include cars and possibly valuable personal possessions, such as a coin collection.

Next go through the list and make sure that someone you trust can manage each asset once your parent is no longer able to do so.

Obviously a power of attorney document can be very helpful in this regard. So too can joint ownership. For example, if your parent has a checking account for paying bills and you become a joint owner of the account, it will make it possible for you to pay all sorts of routine bills without the hassle of constantly trying to get institutions to accept a power of attorney.

You can ask your parent to make you a joint owner of larger assets too, such as investment accounts or even a house. But this arrangement is much more complicated, and you should generally consult an attorney or financial advisor before taking this step. For one thing, making someone a joint owner of a large asset can have unexpected tax consequences. For another, if your parent passes away, the person who is the joint owner will usually immediately become the sole owner, and this outcome might not be exactly what your parent wanted in an estate plan. Also making someone a joint owner can adversely affect planning for Medicaid or other government benefits.

If your parent is still driving, you should be very careful about becoming a joint (or the sole) owner of a car. Doing so could affect your insurance rates and could make you personally liable to anyone your parent injures in a car accident. It's usually better to wait until parents give up driving, and then have them give the car to someone else or donate it to charity (or use your power of attorney to do so).

As Henry David Thoreau once said, "simplify, simplify." Many people's financial lives are unnecessarily complicated, which is especially true of older people in the early stages of dementia. Anything you can do to make your parent's finances simple will be very beneficial. For instance you can consolidate multiple bank accounts and if possible try to have everything in one bank. Old 401(k) accounts can be rolled over into IRAs, and multiple IRAs can be consolidated. Some older people still have paper stock certificates, which can be kept electronically instead. Try to keep all financial records in one place that's easy to access.

You'll also want to gather up your parent's insurance policies. Many people, including those with early dementia, simply allow such policies to renew year after year without thinking about them. Ask yourself if the policy coverage amounts still make sense in your parent's case. Should they be higher or lower? Does your parent still need life insurance? Do the beneficiary designations still make sense? Are the premiums current, or did your parent let a policy lapse?

It's extremely important to find out if parents have purchased long-term care insurance. Such a policy can be very helpful if they eventually need to move to a dementia-care facility. (See Chapter 24 for more information on this type of insurance.)

Speaking of beneficiary designations, you should note that bank accounts, brokerage accounts, and retirement plans typically have such designations that stipulate who will receive the assets if the person dies. It's common for people to fill out such designations when they set up the account and never review their choices again. Forgetting to do so can be a big problem because, in most cases, if the person passes away, the assets in the account will go to whomever is named in the beneficiary designation—*regardless of what the person wrote in a will*. If your parent set up a designation long ago, the assets in the account might well not go to the persons your parent would now prefer. It is important to review this information right away, because it can be hard for someone other than your parent to undo such a designation after the fact.

Make Another Inventory

After you've made an inventory of your parent's assets, it's time to make an inventory of your parent's expenses. What bills does your parent have to pay every month? Are there other, irregular expenses?

It takes some work to pull together such a list, but you'll be amazed at how much easier it is to keep track of everything once you have it. You'll be able to know what bills have been paid each month and which ones are outstanding. You might also be surprised at how many expenses can be eliminated. Many older people have set up automatically recurring charges for services they no longer use, and as dementia sets in, they ignore having them removed. They can include charges for telephone, cable TV, and Internet features that your parent no longer uses, as well as gym memberships, disused home security features, protection plans for appliances and gadgets, credit monitoring services (which may not make sense if your parent is no longer using or applying for credit), automatic donations to charities that your parent no longer understands, and many others.

Again, simplify everything as far as possible. Fewer, easier bills are a godsend. Also because parents with dementia get confused and tend to lose things, it's best to try to reduce the number of your parent's credit cards to one (and preferably zero).

If possible, it's a good idea to start having bills sent to your address (or the address of another trusted person who will handle your parent's finances). Parents with dementia are very good at losing bills and other important documents that arrive in the mail.

More Ways to Protect Your Parent

Here are some other ways to protect your parent financially:

- If your parent regularly receives checks, such as Social Security or pension payments, find out whether you can have them deposited directly into a bank account rather than mailed.

- It's often possible to designate someone other than your parent to receive your parent's real estate tax bills.

- If your parent doesn't have online banking, it's a good idea to set it up, along with online accounts for Social Security, Medicare, and so on. If you set them up with your parent and keep track of passwords and security questions, then in an emergency you can manage finances online. (It's arguably technically illegal to "impersonate" someone else online, but there's no law against helping a parent to accomplish something online. And a power of attorney makes this issue even less of a problem.)

- Your parent can fill out a form called "Authorization to Disclose Personal Health Information" that will allow Medicare to discuss medical and insurance details with you (or anyone else your parent chooses). This form can make it much easier to handle Medicare coverage and payment issues.

- If you're worried about your parent responding to solicitations in the mail, you can ask the post office to discontinue delivery of third-class mail. A number of direct-mail organizations also will let you take your name off mailing lists. (Most mailers would rather save money and *not* mail to people who aren't interested.)

- You can also get your parent's name removed from many telemarketing lists through the website of the U.S. Federal Trade Commission.

- In California you can fill out a document called an "Authorization for Release of Information for Fraud Prevention." This document waives the normal privacy rules and allows a bank to contact you if it notices unusual activity in your parent's account.

• It's a good idea for parents to sign and notarize a form stating that they have dementia and that their signature might change as a result. Having this form can be useful if someone later questions the authenticity of a signature.

If Your Parent Objects

So far our advice in this chapter is based on the assumption that your parent will cooperate in having you or someone else handle financial matters. However, that's not always the case. As with driving, giving up control over finances is a major step that has both symbolic and practical significance. Many parents are reluctant to relinquish control, especially because of the suspiciousness and defensiveness that can result from dementia, and because the nature of the disease itself may prevent parents in the early stages from recognizing that they're not handling their finances as well as they should.

There are often other factors at work too. For instance, many parents (even those who don't have dementia) are simply embarrassed to share the details of their financial life with their children. Many parents (even those who don't have dementia) are reluctant to write wills or other similar documents because they simply don't like to think about the possibility of their own demise. And a number of children are reluctant to bring up the topic of estate planning because they're afraid that it makes them sound greedy.

As a result getting your parent to cooperate with reasonable financial planning can often be a delicate dance. If your parent is married, it can sometimes be easier to get the other spouse to bring up the subject. The spouse can suggest that they both sign powers of attorney "in case something happens to one of us."

Rather than bluntly suggesting that your parent can't manage a checkbook, you might be able to persuade your parent to let you "help out" by taking on "some of the nuisance of paying bills." Many parents are amenable to giving up tasks if they can tell themselves and others that they could do it themselves but they simply don't want to bother.

You can also gently suggest to your parent how much easier it would be to consolidate accounts, reduce the number of credit cards, and otherwise simplify financial matters. You could mention that you've been simplifying your own financial life and offer to help simplify your parent's as well.

If your parent has a financial advisor or similar trusted professional, you might approach that person about making suggestions to your parent. It's often much easier for a parent to take advice from a professional than from a child, simply because it saves face and can be couched as sound financial planning rather than as a sign of mental decline.

If you end up meeting with a lawyer, financial advisor, or other professional along with your parent, and you have questions you don't necessarily want to ask in front of your parent, it's good to let the professional know ahead of time and then have a private conversation later. Parents with early dementia can become highly suspicious if they think that you're talking with someone secretly or behind their back.

Finally if you take over handling your parent's financial affairs, be prepared to have your parent criticize you for not doing it properly. This is extremely common. What's usually behind criticism of this sort is not a mistake on the child's part; it's an attempt by parents to seem relevant and in control, to express frustration at their own inability, and to act as though they still understand everything that's happening. So don't take the criticism personally, because it's not really about you; it's about your parent's frustration over the illness.

14

When Is It Okay to Lie to Your Parent?

One of the difficult issues that almost everyone taking care of a parent with dementia eventually confronts is that occasionally it seems expedient to lie to your parent, or at least not to tell your parent the whole truth. This can create a serious emotional and moral dilemma. Nobody feels like it's simply okay to lie to a parent. Lying can feel wrong and hurtful.

And that's because it *is* wrong and hurtful . . . *if* your parent is normal and healthy. But when a parent has dementia, the calculus changes considerably. Lying should never be a default option obviously, but there are times when not being completely and bluntly truthful can amount to providing sensitive and loving care.

It's worth thinking a bit about this issue before it arises if possible, since it will make you more prepared for dealing with it down the road.

Most commonly the question of whether it's okay to lie comes up in three situations: When a parent is diagnosed with dementia (or you've concluded that he or she has the disease without a formal diagnosis), when you're having trouble getting your parent to do something important, and when your parent is experiencing delusions.

When a Parent Is Diagnosed

People in the early stages of dementia often don't want to admit the extent of their problem. They may be in denial because they're afraid of the disease or of what people will say or what will happen to them. Also the disease itself may prevent them from understanding their condition.

As a result, very often the first "is it okay to lie?" dilemma arises over whether to be honest about the simple fact that a parent has a memory issue. Some family members are afraid to be honest for fear that doing so will make the dementia sufferer scared or depressed.

As it turns out, these fears may be overblown. One scientific study found that receiving a formal dementia diagnosis was very unlikely to cause seniors to become depressed or upset, and in fact it often resulted in *less* anxiety for them because they finally had a clear explanation for the symptoms they had been experiencing.

However, everyone is different (and people with dementia are often different on different days and at different times of the day). For this reason, it's not *always* advisable to be brutally honest about the extent of a parent's condition.

Denial exists as a defense mechanism by which the psyche protects itself against an experience it would find traumatic and debilitating. Therefore in some circumstances confronting people with a hard truth can cause unnecessary trauma—the person might be better able to accept the truth at a later time. Another problem is that it can cause people to become defensive and to push away the truth teller—which could make it harder for you to take care of your parent.

Remember that a good goal for your relationship is to always ask "What's most important?" It's not necessarily important that your parent accept and acknowledge the disease. What's important is that your parent's needs are taken care of.

If the issue comes up, it's often possible to fudge the answer. A comment such as "Well I'm not a doctor, but I think that as you're getting older you're probably tending to forget things a little more often" is completely truthful but avoids providing a diagnosis.

On the other hand, there are situations where doing the most important thing may require a more direct level of honesty. For instance, if you believe that it's dangerous for your parent to drive a car or to manage medications without help, then sidestepping the question may be a very bad idea.

For Your Parent's Own Good

Another dilemma arises when children try to get their parent to do something that is for the parent's own benefit, but the parent refuses because the disease is causing fear, anxiety, or suspicion. Is it okay to stretch the truth in order to get your parent to do something beneficial?

There's no one-size-fits-all answer to this question, but once again it's helpful to ask yourself "What's most important?" As a care partner, you have to pick your battles. It might be nice if parents always undressed before going to bed, for example, but if they spend an occasional night with their clothes on, it's not the end of the world. This might be a fight that's simply not worth having. On the other hand, taking important medication or going to the doctor for a medical test might be something that you think is essential.

In such cases, one way to think about what you're doing is that you're not so much *lying* to your parent as *translating* for him or her. The word *lying* connotes deliberately misleading or tricking people to get away with something or to get them to do something that's against their interests. But that's not at all what you're doing. You're trying to get your parent to do something that your parent would obviously want to do if not for the disease, and you're doing it by translating the situation into a message that he or she can make sense of.

Imagine an accomplished golf instructor teaching a beginner. The instructor might be able to explain in highly complex terms what the beginner is doing wrong, but doing so would only make the student confused and anxious. So the instructor will simply suggest that the beginner do something differently. Instructors often try to get beginners to overcorrect for their mistakes in the hope that, by trying to overcorrect, the beginner will end up doing roughly the right thing. Telling the student to overcorrect is technically lying, since the instructor is not stating exactly what the student should do. But the intent is not to mislead or deceive; the intent is to *translate* the message into a form that will allow the student to be successful in the long run. That's what you're doing with your parent—translating the message in a way that your parent can understand and that will ultimately make him or her happy and safe.

To be sure, there's an art to this. It's not always easy; it's a skill, but it's a skill that can be learned. An important point is that you seldom—and only if absolutely necessary—want to mislead parents in a way that will cause them to stop trusting you. Trust is a linchpin of being able to care for someone. (Of course a perverse advantage of dementia can be that even if in a very difficult situation you do something that your parent considers a violation of trust, he or she might well not remember this fact the next day.)

Another thing to remember is that it's good to listen to feelings, not just words. If your parent is uncooperative, it's generally due to fear or anxiety. Your first line of defense is usually to acknowledge the fear or anxiety and respond in a manner that is loving and reassuring. Stretching the truth is a last, if sometimes necessary, resort.

A final consideration is that you can always ask yourself "If my parent were somehow able—in this one moment—to understand everything that I understand, what would my parent want me to do?" This question may well lead you to the conclusion that your parent would want you to do what's best in the long run.

Delusions

Delusions are a special situation in which not being entirely honest with your parent may be particularly appropriate.

Suppose, for instance, that your mother tells you that she just had a long phone call from her own mother—which is impossible because your grandmother passed away many years ago. Should you tell your mother that she's mistaken? You might think that allowing your mother to believe her delusion amounts to lying on your part, or at least behaving in a misleading way. You might also think that it's good to bring your mother back to reality by telling her the truth.

For many children, their parents' delusions are extremely upsetting—often more upsetting than they are to the parents themselves. That's because delusions bring home in a very dramatic way the extent of the illness and the degree to which the parents are no longer themselves. Many children try to dispel delusions at least as much to make themselves feel better as to make the parent feel better.

But consider this fact: At the moment, your mother genuinely believes that her own mother is alive and well. If you tell her that her mother is dead, it's going to come as an enormous shock. Imagine your own reaction if you suddenly discovered that a close relative had passed away. You'd experience dismay, grief, and misery. Your mother might well react in the same manner. What you might think of in a casual way as dispelling a delusion could in fact be forcing your mother to go through the emotional trauma of losing a close relative all over again.

Many delusions experienced by people with dementia are harmless—they might in fact be pleasant—and they go away after a short time. In the spirit of asking "What's most important," you might find that there is very little to gain and much to lose by being brutally truthful.

So how should you react? It's usually not in fact necessary for you to pass judgment on the truth or falsity of your parent's claims. You could simply change the subject. Or you could ask how your grandmother is and what she said. Asking such questions isn't lying, after all. You could also ask how your mother feels about the phone call, which is to bring the subject back to your parent's feelings in the moment rather than dwelling on the content of the delusions.

There is nothing morally wrong with embracing your parent's experience as your parent's experience. When someone tells us about a dream, for instance, we are usually entertained and don't feel obligated to insist that the events in the dream didn't really happen. Similarly as long as a parent's delusions are harmless, it might well be appropriate simply to ignore or indulge them.

On the other hand, if a parent's delusions are causing significant anxiety or distress, then it might be a good idea to challenge them. The best way to challenge a parent's delusions is often *not* to simply state, "That's not true!" After all, your parent is experiencing the delusion as real. If you flatly deny it, you're creating a situation in which your parent must choose between believing you and believing their own experience. This choice can create a tremendous amount of anxiety, and your parent might react by becoming hostile or suspicious.

Some children respond by trying to prove that the parent is wrong. For instance if the parent believes there's a burglar in the bedroom, the child might open the door and exclaim, "See? No one's there!" But this response can also cause problems, because in a sense it forces the parent to admit being crazy or deluded. Parents will typically try to find a way out of this admission. "Well, he was there a minute ago," they will say. "He must have slipped out the window." The parent is no less anxious about the burglar, but has now also become defensive and antagonistic.

With some unpleasant delusions, it's possible to relieve your parent's anxiety simply through redirection. You can change the subject, offer something pleasant, bring up an interesting piece of news, or suggest a new activity. If you respond in a way that's positive and enthusiastic, your parent might well become involved in the new subject and simply forget about the delusion.

When a parent persists in believing an unpleasant delusion, a good approach might be to express polite doubt and a willingness to work with the parent to investigate. "Really, a burglar?" you might say. "Gee, I didn't notice anything unusual. But let's check it out. . . . Hmmm, there doesn't seem to be anyone in the bedroom. And happily nothing valuable is missing." You *don't* have to draw the conclusion that "there was no burglar"—and therefore that your parent was wrong—you just have to provide facts from which your parent can conclude that there is nothing to worry about. As long as you're just providing evidence and not drawing a conclusion yourself, you're not creating cognitive dissonance or forcing your parent to choose between believing you and believing his or her own senses. (And having relieved your parent's anxiety, it might be a good time to make another attempt at redirection. Your parent might now be happy to change the subject.)

If your parent is persistently experiencing unpleasant delusions, it might be good to talk to a doctor. Sometimes delusions are caused by conditions other than dementia, such as a urinary tract infection, blood sugar fluctuations, or a thyroid abnormality. If the delusions are caused by dementia, you might want to talk with the doctor about antipsychotic medications. These drugs won't necessarily eliminate the delusions, but they might enable your parent to experience less anxiety as a result of them.

15

Keeping Your Parent Safe at Home

For a parent with dementia, living at home can sometimes be dangerous—or at least there are a lot of potential hazards. It's a good idea to inspect your parent's home (or your own home if your parent lives with you) and become aware of ways to reduce these hazards.

If you've raised a child, then you've gone through a similar process before. At some point you undoubtedly childproofed your home to remove anything that could cause a toddler to get hurt. In a similar way, you'll want to "dementia-proof" your home to keep your parent from getting hurt.

In general there are three main safety concerns for a parent with dementia: preventing falls, preventing wandering, and preventing your parent from coming into contact with something that could cause an injury. A final consideration is preventing your parent from losing anything important.

This chapter takes the form of a series of checklists. At first such checklists might seem overwhelming. But don't worry; they are not endless lists of tasks. They're simply a helpful guide that you can use as you walk around your home. Not everything on these lists needs to be done for every person with dementia, and some of them might not be necessary now but might become important later. However, going through the list is a good exercise and can get you thinking about relatively simple ways to make your parent's environment safer.

If you spend an hour or so walking around the house where your parent lives with these lists, deciding which items apply to you and which ones don't, you'll probably end up with your own to-do list of actions you can take that can make your parent safer, and a sense of which ones need to be done right away and which ones can wait. Then you can begin to take care of them and cross them off the list. As with everything else involving dementia, taking a little time now to be proactive can prevent having to deal with a crisis down the road.

Also it might be worth contacting your local elder services agency. Some agencies will send a specialist to do a free home safety check.

Here are the checklists grouped into categories:

Preventing Falls

❑ Loose rugs, such as throw rugs and small area rugs, are a falling hazard. It's best to simply remove them.

❑ Bath mats can also be a hazard. Be sure they have a nonslip surface on the underside.

❑ Check the home for other small items that can be tripping hazards. They include ottomans, magazine racks, floor lamps in some cases, and long extension cords.

❑ Coffee tables can be a danger. They're low enough that many older people don't see them as they're walking. Also, older people often stumble over them as they try to get up from a sofa. Removing them can be a smart idea.

❑ Stairs are an obvious hazard. Having your parent sleep on the first floor if possible can prevent a lot of problems. Some people install baby gates on stairs to keep parents from using them.

❑ Many falls are the result of poor lighting. Simply increasing the wattage of light bulbs in dark areas can help. It's also a good idea to install night-lights anywhere your parent might go during the night. Many night-lights operate on a motion sensor, which makes them a smart choice for bathrooms.

❑ Clutter is another common cause of falls, because it can be tripped over and because it can be confusing to people with moderate-to-severe dementia. Keeping the environment as free of unnecessary clutter as possible is difficult but very helpful.

❑ Outside the house, it's wise to fix chipped or uneven steps, install handrails, repair raised stepping stones, prune bushes that get in the way of walkways, and keep hoses coiled up when not in use. Some people put reflective tape on the edges of steps to make them more visible. You might also want to consider installing a ramp so that your parent doesn't have to climb steps.

❑ If you're concerned that your parent might fall out of bed, you can buy narrow bed guards that will make falling less likely. (You probably don't want full-length bedrails because they can make it very difficult for your parent to get out of bed on purpose and can themselves become a safety hazard.)

Preventing Wandering

Persistent wandering, especially when a parent repeatedly tries to leave the house late at night, is often a concern that persuades families to move a parent to a care facility. However, if your parent has only a slight tendency to wander, there are some steps you can take:

❑ Give your parent an ID bracelet with your address and an emergency phone number. You can also put this information in your parent's purse or wallet.

❑ A more high-tech solution is to give your parent a wearable device, such as a watch, that's equipped with GPS. If your parent goes wandering, you'll be able to track his or her location.

❑ A baby monitor can alert you when your parent is up at night. You can also use motion-sensor alarms for this purpose. And you can install alarms on windows and doors that will let you know if your parent is trying to leave.

❑ Some families put large "Stop" signs on exterior doors or other places where they don't want a parent to go. In many cases, this is surprisingly effective.

Preventing Injuries

Going through your house and looking for hazardous items that could cause injuries is very similar to childproofing a home for toddlers. The most important areas to consider are the kitchen, bathrooms, laundry room, and garage.

KITCHEN

❑ Kitchen ranges can be a fire hazard, especially if there's any chance your parent could try to heat food and then forget it's there. If you don't want to completely unplug the stove, other options include installing a hidden gas valve that you can operate but that your parent is unlikely to be able to locate, using safety knobs, and adding a timer that will automatically shut the range off after a certain amount of time. An electrician should be able to help you with these items; you can also contact the range's manufacturer.

❑ Consider locking up knives, matches, cleaning supplies, alcohol, scissors, and plastic bags. You can buy a child safety cabinet latch for this purpose.

❑ You might want to disconnect the garbage disposal or ask a plumber to make it more difficult to use.

❑ Get rid of decorative fruits and vegetables, food-shaped magnets, and other items that your parent might mistake for food.

BATHROOMS

❑ While there are limits to how many changes you can make in a bathroom, walk-in showers and grab bars are ideal. Easier changes to make include getting a bath stool and a raised toilet seat.

❑ Lock up any medicines that you normally keep in the medicine cabinet.

❑ Remove or lock up cleaning supplies. As in the kitchen, consider putting a child safety latch on vanity cabinets.

❑ Use plastic cups rather than glasses that could break.

❑ Put a foam rubber cover over the bathtub faucet to help prevent injuries if your parent falls in the tub. These are often available as a child safety item.

❑ Install a water temperature regulator, or simply lower the temperature on the water heater—a maximum of 120 degrees Fahrenheit (or 50 degrees Celsius) is good.

❑ Install automatic faucet control devices. These are small wands that extend from the faucet; the water flows only when you touch them.

These devices prevent parents from leaving the water on indefinitely and possibly causing overflows and water damage.

❑ Consider removing or locking up hair dryers, which can be an electrical hazard.

LAUNDRY ROOM

❑ If possible, simply lock the laundry room.

❑ If you can't lock the room, keep laundry detergent locked up or otherwise secure (again, you might want to use a child-safety latch).

❑ Consider putting safety locks on the washer and dryer so your parent can't open them.

GARAGE

❑ Garages often contain a lot of unsafe items. If possible, simply lock the garage.

❑ If you can't lock the garage, try to lock up the following items, put them on high shelves, or otherwise make them inaccessible: lawn mowers, weed trimmers, lawn care supplies, fertilizer, mothballs, toxic cleaners, power tools, gasoline, paint, fuel for grilling, fishing tackle, sports equipment, and bicycles.

❑ With larger items, such as lawn mowers and bicycles, if you can't otherwise secure them, try to cover them so they're not obvious.

OTHER AREAS

❑ Remove locks on bathroom doors (and doors to other rooms) that could result in your parent becoming locked in a room and unable to figure out how to escape.

❑ Add security locks to high windows and balconies.

❑ Be very cautious with portable space heaters and electric blankets.

❑ If your parent smokes, encourage quitting. At the very least, lock up or hide matches and lighters. Many parents with dementia simply forget about the desire to smoke if cigarettes are not available. Your parent's doctor might also be able to recommend medications that will reduce cravings.

❑ Remove guns from the house.

❑ Tape stickers or decals to glass doors and large windows at eye level if you think your parent might walk into them.

❑ Insert child-safety plugs into unused electrical outlets.

❑ Remove any plants that would be toxic if eaten. (If you're in doubt, contact a nursery or poison control center.)

❑ Fish tanks can sometimes be dangerous; it's often best to remove them or place them out of reach.

❑ If you have a pool, lock the gate or otherwise find ways to prevent your parent from falling into it. (If possible, you might want to ask any neighbors who have pools to do the same.)

❑ Make a list of emergency phone numbers (including the fire department, poison control center, and the like) and keep it on your phone and in a prominent place.

❑ Consider hiding a spare house key in the yard in case your parent accidentally locks you out.

Preventing Losing Things

❑ Hide, remove, or lock up valuables, including cash, silver, expensive jewelry, and important documents.

❑ Always check wastebaskets before emptying them to see if your parent threw away something important. (It's not uncommon for parents to put dentures or hearing aids in a napkin and then throw away the napkin, for example.)

❑ Get spare sets of all keys.

❑ You can buy small electronic "key finders" that can be attached to key rings; if the keys are lost, you can use your smartphone to make the device issue a loud sound. You might be able to attach such devices to other important (and easy-to-lose) items, such as eyeglasses and TV remotes.

16

Getting Help When Your Parent Lives at Home or with You

If you're taking care of a parent with dementia who lives in his or her own home or with you, the tasks and responsibilities can be overwhelming. It would be great if you could take care of everything yourself—and many people mistakenly believe that they *should* do it all themselves—but the reality is that, at some point, it simply becomes impossible. Eventually people with dementia require round-the-clock care, which no human being can provide.

Thus, it makes sense at some point to start getting some outside help. Most people begin by turning to family and friends, and in some cases family members can be remarkably helpful and supportive. But family and friends are not always available, and even when they are, some types of help require skills or training that family members simply don't have.

The good news is that a wide variety of outside services are available. They usually cost money of course, but some are available at reduced cost, and it's generally possible to use them in a relatively cost-effective way.

How to Think about Outside Services

If you're going to use outside services effectively, it's important to think about them in the right way.

First of all, using outside services is not an admission of weakness or failure. It's a sign of thoughtful and effective caregiving. When you're caring for a parent with dementia, the principal resource you have to offer is *time*. And your time is not infinite. The tasks you have to do might seem infinite, but the time you have available is not.

So it's a good idea to apply the goal of asking "What's most important?" What are the best choices you can make with the necessarily limited time you have available? What are the tasks that only *you* can do to make your parent happy and comfortable? For example, anyone can mow your parent's lawn, but only you can reminisce about happy childhood memories. When possible, therefore, it makes sense to hire a neighborhood teenager to mow the lawn and spend your time reminiscing.

A good way to think of yourself is as a business manager who is outsourcing or delegating tasks. The reason good managers delegate tasks is *not* because they can't do them themselves, but because delegating allows them to be more efficient, to get more accomplished, and to focus their time on the tasks that have the greatest value. In the same way, delegating tasks to outside services allows you to be more efficient and to take better care of your parent.

When deciding what tasks to delegate, the following are good candidates:

- *Menial tasks,* such as housecleaning, lawn mowing, shopping, errands, routine meal preparation, and so on. These chores take a lot of time but don't tremendously enrich your parent's life, and they're chores that other people can usually do reasonably well.

- *Tasks you can't do because of conflicting commitments,* such as looking after a parent while you're at work.

- *Specialized tasks,* such as occupational therapy.

- *Tasks that others can do much more efficiently.* For instance, it might be worth hiring a mover for an hour to rearrange heavy furniture, rather than trying to do it yourself.

"They Won't Do It Right"

Some caregivers object to the idea of using an outside service on the grounds that someone else won't do the task correctly, or at least won't do it in exactly the same way. And that's true—someone else *won't* do the task in exactly the same way. A housecleaner will clean differently from the way you do. But the question is "What's most important?" A good way to think about it is not to ask whether the task was accomplished perfectly, but whether the *difference* in how well it was accomplished is worth the time and stress you saved as a result. Unless your housecleaner is utterly incompetent, you'll generally find that having less to do and worry about is well worth putting up with having things taken care of a little differently.

A more frequent experience is that *your parent* will object to having someone else perform certain tasks. It's extremely common for parents to complain that outside service providers don't do them in the right way. Sometimes they will tell you that the outside provider was rude or even that the person stole something.

You don't want to reject such accusations completely out of hand, but it's worth noting that in an enormous number of cases what's causing parents' objections is not a genuine shortcoming on the part of a service provider but simply the parent's fear. Parents with dementia have difficulty comprehending and adapting to change. They might not immediately understand why someone new is doing something in their home—even if you've explained it to them many times. They might be afraid that you're not going to be there for them or that they're being abandoned.

This is a serious problem, but it's no reason not to hire a service provider. Remember, you're hiring a provider in order to take *better* care of your parent. While the provider might cause your parent some initial discomfort, in the long run delegating is going to make your parent feel happier and better taken care of.

Plan Ahead

As with everything else involving dementia care, planning ahead is key. It's a good idea to start investigating and lining up service providers before you need them—because eventually you will, and by that point you'll be under a lot more stress. Scouting providers ahead of time means that you'll make much better decisions when the time comes.

If you don't think it will upset your parent, you might want to discuss the fact that you might eventually need some help. It's unlikely that your parent will remember this discussion later on, but doing so can help you to feel better about the decision.

What follows is an overview of some of the types of services that are available. Some services are specially designed for dementia sufferers; others are for older people who need help in general; and some are simply intended to make life easier for anyone who is busy. More detailed information on finding these services can be found in the Resources at the back of the book. For now it's worth thinking about the broad range of available services and which types of tasks you can delegate in order to make your life easier and focus your time on activities of greatest value to you and your parent.

Adult Day Centers

Adult day centers provide care, companionship, activities, and social interaction for seniors. Some have special units for people with dementia, and some focus entirely on people with dementia.

Adult day centers are similar in some ways to day care, except that they serve adults rather than children. If you're working while taking care of a parent, day centers can provide a safe place for your parent to be while you're at work. They can also provide social activities and mental stimulation for your parent while giving you regular opportunities to run errands or get some rest and relaxation.

There are more than 5,600 adult day centers in the United States, and almost 80 percent of them operate on a nonprofit basis. The average age of participants is 72, and about two-thirds are women. One study found that slightly more than half of all participants have some form of cognitive impairment.

Although they're typically called day centers, some also have evening hours. Many offer meals and some provide transportation. Some offer health services, including help with medications, blood pressure checks, eye and ear exams, dental cleanings, and podiatrist visits. Some offer counseling and physical therapy. A number of day centers provide access to a barber or hairdresser and help with laundry.

Some centers offer more focused and intensive health and therapy services for people who might otherwise be at risk of needing a nursing home. They are often called adult day health care centers.

Because dementia can make people wary of change, many parents resist the idea of going to day centers, and may seem to dislike them at first. But if a center is well run, over time parents usually become used to it and often end up enjoying the activities and social interaction.

It's common for centers to offer a trial period, such as a week, before asking you to sign up for a longer term.

When choosing an adult day center, you'll want to ask about activities, meals, transportation, costs and fees, and hours. A visit to the center will give you an opportunity to observe what actually happens during the day and how the staff members interact with participants.

Some other good questions to ask include:

- Is the center a for-profit or nonprofit one? Is it connected to a government agency, religious organization, or health care facility?

- What types of medical services are available?

- How long has the center been operating?

- What credentials do the staff members have? Is there a registered nurse and/or a certified social worker on staff? If not, is there one on call?

- What's the ratio of staff members to participants? (The national average is one staff member for every six participants. Many U.S. states have established staff-ratio requirements, which vary from 1:4 to 1:10.)

- Are there provisions for seniors with mobility problems, disabilities, or incontinence issues?

- If the center offers meals, can it accommodate special dietary needs?

- If your parent is signed up on a weekly or monthly basis but misses a day for health problems or other reasons, will you get a refund?

Medicare does not pay for adult day centers, but some private insurance might. Medicaid sometimes pays for adult day centers through Home and Community-Based Services waivers, also known as 1915(c) waivers—especially if the alternative is that the person would be put into a nursing home. There are often waiting lists for these waivers, however. Some state Medicaid programs offer more limited benefits that can be used while waiting for a full waiver. Some states also have a separate nursing home diversion program designed to help people avoid a nursing home by using an adult day healthcare center instead.

In the United States, certain veterans' pensions, such as Aid and Attendance, will pay for adult day care, as will Veterans Directed Care programs. The VHA Medical Benefits package won't pay for adult day care, but it will pay for adult day health care if you can show that it's necessary for medical reasons. The percentage of the cost that the package covers depends on your financial situation.

Respite Care

Even if you don't want to sign up your parent for a regular weekly or monthly schedule at an adult day center, you might occasionally want to use one for a brief time simply so that you can take a break. This type of occasional short-term caregiving is called *respite care*.

Many adult day centers offer respite care. Some assisted-living facilities and dementia-care facilities also offer a respite option, in which your parent can live in the facility for a short time without moving in permanently. And many home-care agencies will arrange for someone to provide in-home respite care wherever your parent lives.

Respite care is ideal if you need someone to look after your parent while you take a vacation or are busy with unavoidable commitments, or if you simply need time off to avoid burnout.

Respite care can also be a good way of introducing your parent to the idea of an adult day center or live-in facility. Parents might be much less resistant to the idea of going to such a facility if they know that it's only for a short time, and the resulting familiarity can make for a smoother transition later.

Even if you don't need a respite option at the moment, it's a good idea to begin researching respite care now. That's because a situation could arise suddenly in which you won't be able to take care of your parent for a while, and you'll need to quickly make other arrangements. If you've done your homework ahead of time, it will be much easier to handle such a situation should it occur.

In-Home Services

Many discrete services—less comprehensive than respite care—can be provided in your parent's home. These services tend to fall into two groups, depending on whether the provider is a skilled health care professional.

Skilled in-home health care includes nurses and others with special training who come to your parent's home to handle medical needs, such as wound care or injections, or to provide physical, speech, or occupational therapy. In most cases, you won't need to hire someone for this purpose yourself; the services will be provided or coordinated by a home health care agency after authorization by your parent's doctor.

Medicare typically covers these costs, as long as they're medically necessary and your parent can't easily go to a health care facility.

Other types of services, which you'll typically have to arrange and pay for yourself, include:

Personal-care services, such as help with eating, bathing, dressing, toileting, exercise, and other types of personal care and hygiene.

Homemaker services, including general housekeeping, meal preparation, and shopping.

Companionship services provided by people who visit patients with dementia, keep them company, and engage in recreational activities.

While you can certainly hire individuals directly to provide these types of services, it can be preferable to go through a home-care agency. One advantage is that an agency can provide substitute help on short notice if a provider gets sick. Agencies also typically perform background checks on employees and can be held responsible if an employee damages something in your home or is injured on your property.

When interviewing individuals for these services, good questions to ask include whether they have experience with dementia care and whether they're trained in first aid and CPR. You should also ask for references and follow up by contacting them.

When a parent has very early-stage dementia, it's not as essential that an in-home provider have specialized dementia training. However, as the disease progresses and your parent begins to have more serious communication and behavioral issues in addition to occasional memory lapses, specialized dementia training and experience become essential so that the provider can handle unexpected situations.

When you begin working with an in-home service provider, it's a good idea to take a few minutes and talk with the person in some detail about your parent. You can explain your parent's level of cognition and also describe his or her personality, history, likes and dislikes, as well as favorite memories, hobbies, or topics of conversation. Sharing this information with the provider can smooth the transition and help your parent to adjust to having the provider around.

You can also give the provider any special instructions—for instance, a homemaker should be very careful emptying the trash if your parent might have accidentally thrown away jewelry, hearing aids, dentures, and so on.

Meal Delivery and Transportation

For parents with early dementia—who are having trouble with cooking but not eating—meal-delivery services, such as Meals on Wheels, can be an excellent option. They're a way to make sure your parent has regular healthy meals without always having to cook them yourself or worry that your parent will become injured trying to use the kitchen.

Many grocery stores also offer online ordering and delivery. While your parent might not be able to handle the ordering or putting all the food away, it can be a convenience for you since it saves a trip to the grocery store.

Transportation can be scary for people with dementia, and unfortunately there are very few services that provide safe transportation for dementia sufferers.

If your parent is in a wheelchair, you can hire a chair car. Ridesharing services, such as Uber and Lyft, sometimes offer the option of wheelchair-accessible rides. If your parent has very advanced dementia and absolutely needs to travel for medical reasons, often the best option is an ambulance, which can typically be arranged through your parent's regular health care provider.

Professional Care Managers

In response to the growing number of seniors who need care, and particularly care for dementia, a new profession has developed: the geriatric care manager. These managers can perform a range of duties from arranging and coordinating outside services to making ongoing assessments of a senior's condition and tailored recommendations for health, financial, and safety issues.

Many care managers work for an institution such as a hospital, assisted-living facility, nursing home, or hospice agency. However, they can also be hired privately to help coordinate care. As your parent's needs increase, it can be helpful to consult with a care manager, who can make recommendations for outside services and other ways to improve your parent's situation (and your own). Another advantage of using a care manager is that an outside professional can sometimes help to resolve difficult disputes among siblings or other family members as to what type of care your parent truly needs.

The Aging Life Care Association (ALCA; *www.aginglifecare.org*) is a professional association for geriatric care managers. Members who hold an advanced-level membership have a college degree, 3 years of supervised experience (or 2 years plus a degree in a specifically related field), and an ALCA certification.

A group called the National Council of Certified Dementia Practitioners (NCCDP; *www.nccdp.org*) specializes in dementia care. Certified NCCDP members must be registered or licensed practical nurses or have bachelor's degrees in health care, have completed an advanced dementia training program, and have 3 years of experience working directly with dementia sufferers and 1 year of experience in a management role.

17

How to Take Away the Car Keys

Driving a car requires coordination, concentration, orientation, perception, memory, and processing information quickly. In other words, it requires the very same abilities that dementia attacks. At some point, every person who suffers from dementia long enough will become unable to safely operate a motor vehicle.

Unfortunately there's no clear test for exactly when that point arrives. Some people with mild dementia symptoms are able to retain good driving skills for a while, although others are not. Everyone, however, will at some point need to give up driving.

Doing so is easier for some people than for others. There are some parents with dementia who have a good sense that they are losing their skills and who voluntarily relinquish their car keys, although not nearly as many as would be ideal.

Sometimes parents simply start curtailing their driving. For instance, they might choose to avoid driving at night, in bad weather, on busy highways, or at times when there is a lot of traffic. They won't necessarily admit (to themselves or others) that it's because of dementia. They might blame a vision problem. They might complain that traffic in the area has become much worse lately, and that they can no longer stand it. This is fine—the important thing is not that they admit to their disease; it's that they stop endangering themselves and others.

Nevertheless many people—even those who have curtailed their driving—refuse to take the final step and give up their keys. And some are in complete denial (or are unable, owing to the disease, to understand their increasing lack of ability) and insist on continuing to drive even when driving is clearly hazardous or even after several accidents or near accidents.

What can you do?

There's no easy solution, but the first step is to realize that—as with finances—you may need to be proactive about the matter. You can't simply ignore it or assume that your parent will do the right thing. It's possible, but the odds may well be against it, and the stakes are high.

Start Early

In early dementia, it can be a good idea to lay the groundwork for the eventual need to give up driving. You can talk about the fact that your parent will *eventually* have to do so. Placing it in an indeterminate future can make it easier for your parent to contemplate the possibility. Your parent might even agree to give up driving if certain things happen. Of course that doesn't mean that your parent will honor the agreement when the time comes—or even remember it—but it can be a lot easier for you to take away the car keys if you can honestly say that you're not simply imposing your will, but rather executing a plan that your parent made in the past.

When having this discussion, it's best to try to avoid being adversarial. If you come across as the enemy of your parent's freedom, it's bound to create defensiveness. A good attitude is that you're on your parent's side, and the two of you together are making plans regarding how to cope with a common enemy, which is the disease (or, if your parent won't acknowledge the disease, simply with getting older).

You might also want to consider—and perhaps discuss—alternatives to driving. For a great many people, driving represents freedom and autonomy. It symbolizes their ability to go where they want, do as they please, and not be dependent on others. Not being able to drive conjures up images of being trapped as a prisoner in one's own home, never being able to go anywhere, and being totally dependent on other people for the necessities of life.

Therefore anything you can do to persuade your parent that this isn't the case—and to make it not the case—will likely ease the decision to give up having a car.

The good news is that today there are more services than ever before to help people who don't drive. It's often possible to order groceries and have them delivered. Some barbers and hairdressers will make home visits. Many dry cleaners deliver. A number of errand services are available to handle minor tasks for a reasonable fee. It's worth briefly looking into these services ahead of time so you can describe them to your parent.

Many public transit services now offer special rides for the elderly. And ride-sharing services, such as Uber, may be very helpful because they don't require seniors to use money, don't have a fixed schedule, and offer door-to-door service.

Of course you or your relatives might be willing to give your parent a ride as needed. Some parents strongly prefer to be driven by someone they know and trust—but on the other hand, some feel overly dependent as a result and prefer to use alternative services for as long as possible. You might want to ask early on which way of getting around your parent would prefer.

The goal of this discussion is to make parents feel that their freedom is not completely at stake—that they can give up driving and still have a measure of autonomy and choice.

When the Time Comes

At some point you will become convinced that your parent is no longer safe behind the wheel. If your parent refuses to stop driving, what steps can you take?

You could of course simply confiscate your parent's car keys. However, this isn't always the best solution. Your parent might become furious. And if your parent is furious at you or not speaking to you, it could be next to impossible to provide care in other ways. Also it might not even solve the problem—some parents in this situation have managed to borrow or rent a car and continue driving anyway.

If you feel that your parent shouldn't be driving but you want to avoid a confrontation, one possibility is to get someone else to play the "villain." For instance, your parent's doctor might be willing to order your parent not to drive. If your parent is defensive about accepting a diagnosis of dementia, the doctor might be able to blame the order on some other problem, such as difficulty with vision or a physical issue that limits flexibility or coordination. Many parents are much more amenable to giving up driving if they can tell friends and family that they gave it up as a result of a physical ailment rather than because of dementia. (For that matter, some parents are able to save face by saying that they had to give up their car because it no longer worked—so if you're willing to stretch the truth a bit, you can tell your parent that his or her car failed an inspection.)

If your doctor orders your parent not to drive, it can be a good idea to get the order in writing so you can produce it if your parent forgets about it. Another alternative is for the doctor to refer your parent for an independent driving evaluation. In the United States, evaluations are typically offered through the state motor vehicle department. An evaluator will take your parent for a driving test, and if your suspicions about impairment are correct, your parent's license will be suspended. Many parents in this situation will still be furious—but the advantage is that they will be furious at the evaluator, not at you, so your relationship with your parent won't be harmed.

If a doctor doesn't want to refer your parent for a driving test, another option is to contact the local police department or your parent's automobile insurance company and ask them to make a referral (keeping your name out of it if possible).

In some states, doctors who diagnose someone with dementia are legally required to notify the state motor vehicle department. A diagnosis of mild dementia may trigger an evaluation; a diagnosis of moderate or severe dementia may result in an automatic license suspension.

Not all doctors are comfortable with addressing the driving issue. Many primary care doctors in particular simply leave it to families to work out. A memory-care specialist—such as a geriatrician, neurologist, or geriatric psychiatrist—might be more willing to confront the issue directly.

Other Ideas

If your parent is hell-bent on driving despite any medical or legal restrictions, you might want to disable the car. One way to do this is to disconnect the battery cables. There are some downsides to this method, including the fact that it can be tricky to do it correctly and you won't be able to move the car in an emergency.

A simpler idea is to replace your parent's car key with a fake key. Most cars today require a key with a chip in order to start the vehicle. You can often get a copy of a key made without a chip for very little money. Such a key will fit into the ignition but will not start the car. To your parent, it will seem like the car has a mechanical problem.

You can also ask a mechanic to install a hidden *kill switch* in the car. This is a switch that must be activated in order for the car to run. The advantage is that you can still operate the car normally, but your parent can't do so unless he or she finds and figures out the switch. Some families simply remove the car and tell the dementia sufferer that it's in the repair shop.

If you can eventually get your parent to voluntarily give up driving, it can be helpful to provide a lot of praise for making such a wise decision. After all, it's not easy to do. Rewarding parents with compliments and affirmation for caring about other people's safety might make them feel better about the decision and less likely to have second thoughts.

Of course only you can tell whether this is a good suggestion. With some parents, this type of praise might only serve to remind them of their lack of mobility.

As a final thought, it's usually not a good idea to tempt parents who have recently given up driving by leaving your car keys in plain sight or talking unnecessarily about your own driving.

18

What Causes Problem Behaviors

Anyone who has taken care of a person with dementia understands that dementia sufferers often have *problem behaviors*. At a minimum, they can be stubborn, uncooperative, and difficult. They can also become argumentative, aggressive, verbally abusive, and destructive. And they can do things that are highly inappropriate and embarrassing.

Parents with dementia might suddenly refuse to eat, bathe, or get dressed. They might blame you for something that isn't your fault or accuse you of trying to hurt them. They might accuse other people of stealing from them or plotting against them. They might cause a scene or suddenly start swearing or using racial slurs that they never used before. They might become aggressive or violent or break things. They might act in ways that are highly sexually inappropriate. They might undress in public. And these behaviors often seem to happen for no reason and at the worst possible time.

Virtually every family of a dementia sufferer has horror stories about the person's behavior. Years later some of these stories may seem amusing in retrospect, but they're almost never funny at the time.

It will never be possible to eliminate these behaviors. But it's possible to some extent to be proactive in preventing them, and it's possible to react to them constructively and in ways that minimize the harm.

This is tremendously important to any dementia-care provider. While taking care of an elderly person is always a lot of work, problematic behaviors tend to be what is most responsible for family members' burnout and for seniors being transferred to a specialized dementia-care facility. Anything you can do to reduce problem behaviors will make it possible for your parent to be cared for in a home environment for a longer time.

The first step in dealing with problem behaviors is to understand what causes them.

It should be noted that occasionally the root of a problem behavior is only indirectly related to dementia—medication side effects, for instance, or a concurrent mental illness, such as depression, or even a highly distracting or stressful environment. Most of the time though the disease of dementia is the reason. And in general, where the disease is the culprit, problem behaviors stem from one of three main causes: confusion, unmet needs, and delusions.

Confusion

The essence of dementia is that people are confused. They can't remember how to do simple tasks that they want to do. They can't keep up with social situations. They are told to do something, but they don't always know why. They may not understand where they are, who is around them, or what is happening. Feeling confused leads to a variety of reactions, all of which are understandable if you can imagine being in such a position.

FRUSTRATION

Not being able to do a simple task, such as finding a program on TV or preparing a meal, can be intensely frustrating. It's doubly frustrating if there's no clear cause to blame it on. For instance, if you realize that you forgot to buy eggs, that's frustrating, but you can at least recognize the specific thing that's bothering you—having made a mistake at the store. But if you take eggs out of the refrigerator and then can't remember how to cook them, that's even more frustrating because there's no one action or decision or mistake that you can focus your frustration on.

Dementia sufferers often deal with this kind of unfocused frustration by aiming it somewhere else. They might complain that the eggs are bad or that the stove doesn't work. Or they might displace their frustration onto some other random, unrelated person or object. What starts out as frustration about an inability to do one task turns into a kind of diffuse antagonism about completely different issues.

This reaction seems illogical, but keep in mind that people in this position aren't able to comprehend and express the source of their feelings.

They just know that they feel upset and frustrated, and it needs to come out somewhere. If they can get angry at someone or something else, at least they can deal with the difficult emotions they're experiencing.

FEAR

If you're confused about what's happening around you, it's normal to feel fear. Fear is a common reaction to any situation that seems unfamiliar and uncertain. People who are afraid of certain activities or situations often try to avoid them. And that's frequently what's happening when dementia sufferers become stubborn and uncooperative. They won't necessarily say it, but they're refusing to do whatever it is you want them to do because they're afraid.

The reason this can be difficult to perceive is that, for a healthy person, it's hard to imagine that someone could actually be fearful of taking a bath, of going to a store, or of some other mundane activity. This is usually compounded by the fact that the person is unlikely (or unable) to express the fact of being afraid. So the person's behavior looks for all the world like inexplicable stubbornness.

It can be as though a person with a phobia refuses to acknowledge it. Imagine a spouse who has a fear of flying but won't admit it and simply balks at every plan for a family vacation. The family will think that he or she is just being troublesome and uncooperative when the real culprit is an unexpressed fear.

Another way in which fear manifests itself is separation anxiety. Dementia sufferers are often afraid of not having a trusted care partner around them. As a result, they become clingy, follow the care partner around constantly, or find excuses to get upset or cause problems if the person is about to go away for a while. The real source of the problem is the fear of being left alone or with unfamiliar people.

SUSPICION

Most people have a natural self-protective instinct. As children, they're taught not to get into a car with strangers. As adults, they're wary of phone scams, too-good-to-be-true offers, and other forms of manipulation. They have a sense that they shouldn't trust people unless they have some basis for trusting them. This natural instinct doesn't completely go away when people develop dementia—but the constant confusion caused by the disease means that they no longer always understand who or what can be trusted. The result is a kind of paranoia—a natural self-protective instinct that's taken to an unfortunate extreme and applied to situations where it's not appropriate.

It's easy for a healthy care partner to perceive that a family member or aide is merely giving someone a bath, making sure the person takes medicine, or writing a check to pay a bill. But to a confused dementia sufferer, it might not be clear that the person isn't a threat or someone who means them harm.

Suspicion can also stem from a desire to make sense of a loss. For instance, if a parent can't find a purse or a sweater and can't comprehend that it might have been left in the refrigerator or some other inappropriate place, it might be easy to conclude that someone stole it. It can be more comforting for parents to believe that people around them are stealing from them than to accept that they're confused and can no longer keep track of things.

DESIRE TO ESCAPE

When people feel confused by a situation, it's a natural instinct to want to escape—to get back to some other situation that they can comprehend. This feeling explains the common tendency of dementia sufferers to wander. Wandering is partly due to confusion—to not understanding where to go and getting lost—but it can also be due to a desire to get away from surroundings that are too difficult to handle.

Many dementia sufferers are obsessed with a desire to go "home." Home could mean an actual previous home, a childhood home, or an imaginary home. But the term *home* for them usually refers in some sense to an environment where they understand the surroundings and don't feel so confused.

Unmet Needs

People with dementia might be physically uncomfortable, or hungry, or want to engage in some activity, or have some other problem, but because of their disease they're not able to express exactly what's wrong and what they need. As a result, they often become cranky and unpleasant and try to get attention in the hope that someone will understand

and help them. They're not being unpleasant in order to be unpleasant; they're acting out to call attention to themselves in the hope of obtaining assistance.

As a result, a good response to problem behaviors is often to try to figure out what the person might need. One of the most important needs that dementia sufferers have is an environment that is not overly stressful. For someone with dementia, it can be taxing to deal with the simplest elements of everyday life. Anything that adds to the stress can be very difficult—including changes in the environment, conversational demands and expectations, loud noises, intense interactions, busy television programs, and too much variety or clutter. Too much stimulation can create a need for downtime so the person can relax, although it can be very difficult for the person to articulate that.

On the other hand, parents with dementia also need a certain amount of mental stimulation and physical activity, and since they're not usually very good at meeting these needs themselves, they can be subject to boredom. A great many problem behaviors occur simply because the parent is bored and has an unmet need for engaging in some sort of activity.

Delusions

Delusions are incorrect perceptions of reality. They're common in dementia, and they can result in problematic behaviors. Ironically the behaviors wouldn't necessarily be all that problematic *if the delusions were accurate*; the behaviors are often just very rational reactions to very irrational ideas.

Take, for instance, a parent who stays up all night because he believes that a burglar is in the house, or a parent who packs all her belongings into suitcases because she believes that she's going on a long trip the next day. These behaviors might be perfectly appropriate if the parent's beliefs were correct; the problem is that they're not.

Related to delusions is *disinhibition*—the tendency of dementia sufferers to lose the part of the brain that censors their behavior and that enables them to behave in socially appropriate ways. This is not really a delusion, except in the sense that the person has an incorrect perception of reality with regard to what is socially expected.

Imagine an elderly person who comes to feel that it's appropriate to walk around naked, swear like a sailor, and be sexually forward with much younger members of the opposite sex. These are not necessarily problem behaviors as far as the dementia sufferer is concerned—the person might very much enjoy them—but they can be extremely embarrassing and humiliating for family members.

In general parents with dementia don't engage in problem behaviors because they've suddenly become ornery, pigheaded, obnoxious, or lewd—however much it might seem like it at the moment to an exasperated family member. Parents exhibit problem behaviors because they flow directly from the symptoms and difficulties inherent in the disease.

Understanding the reasons for these problem behaviors is key—because if you can see what causes them, it's a lot easier to take steps to prevent them and to cope with them when they happen.

Delirium

A specific type of problem behavior is related to *delirium*, a condition to which people with dementia are particularly susceptible. Delirium is a specific mental state. Parents might be experiencing delirium if they're not just more upset, uncooperative, or disinhibited than usual but instead have a sudden and uncharacteristic personality change.

People with *hyperactive* delirium can be very alert and confrontational. They may become highly disoriented, have rapid mood swings, hallucinate, and experience paranoia. On the other hand, people with *hypoactive* delirium can become abnormally withdrawn and sleepy. There is also something called *mixed* delirium, in which the person alternates between the two.

Delirium isn't just a problem behavior; it's a medical condition. It's often caused by a lack of sleep, drug side effects, dehydration, or a urinary tract infection. If you think your parent has delirium, you'll want to speak to a doctor right away, because it can be treated and because people with delirium can be a danger to themselves and others.

The next two chapters discuss strategies for reducing problem behaviors and dealing with them when they occur.

19

How to Reduce Problem Behaviors

You can never eliminate *all* problem behaviors in people with dementia. That's impossible. But there are ways that you can prevent *some* problem behaviors and minimize the intensity of the ones that occur. As with nearly everything else involving caring for a dementia sufferer, being proactive is the key to success. It's far easier to prevent a difficult or destructive behavior than it is to cope with it once it happens.

The previous chapter showed how a great many problem behaviors stem from confusion on the part of the dementia sufferer, resulting in frustration, fear, suspicion, and a desire to escape. Thus the key to preventing or minimizing difficult behaviors is to change the environment and your parent's daily routine in ways that can reduce confusion. Changing your parent's surroundings and routine can also reduce stress, make it easier to navigate situations, and avoid boredom and other types of unmet needs.

Structure the Environment

All of us respond to our environment. Certain rooms or places just make us feel happier than others, for instance. And dementia sufferers are no different. So anything you can do to make the surroundings more reassuring and less confusing is likely to be helpful.

Clutter, for instance, can be highly confusing and can provoke anxiety, so simplifying the environment by eliminating clutter can be helpful. So can making sure that items are kept in the same place all the time so they're easier to find.

While some background music can be soothing, loud noises and the sound of televisions in the background can be hard to process and can create anxiety.

Small ways of adjusting the environment can make a big difference. For instance, parents with early dementia who are starting to have trouble managing their medications might benefit from a pill organizer. It's possible to buy simplified cell phones and TV remotes with large buttons and only the most essential controls. Another helpful device is a *dementia clock* with a large display that has not only the time but also other information spelled out, such as the year, date, day of the week, and whether it's morning, afternoon, evening, and so on.

Labels are also useful. Using sticky notes to label food items in the refrigerator can prevent confusion. You can also use these notes to put reminders in helpful places.

Some parents become upset when they can't find items that they used to need—car keys, wallets, credit cards, and so on. If your parent can no longer manage them, one option is to provide fake ones. You can leave out nonworking car keys, fake credit cards, and play money or a very small amount of real money. Many parents are calmed down by having these essential items handy even if they never use them.

Overall the goal is to make the environment as easy to navigate and stress free as possible. Reducing confusion and anxiety will help reduce problem behaviors.

Structure the Day

In the same way that it's useful to structure space, it's also useful to structure time. A chief problem that dementia sufferers have is that they can't structure the day themselves, which leads to fear and frustration. In general therefore the more you can create structure in a parent's day and keep the structure of activities consistent from one day to the next, the better your parent will be able to manage.

Some care partners worry that their parent will get bored. Of course sometimes parents do experience understimulation, and it's certainly advisable to have an outing or to do something special occasionally. But in general structure and repetition are not boring to people with dementia; they're reassuring. Change of any sort is always a challenge.

Many people with dementia experience *sundowning*, which refers to the fact that their symptoms get worse toward evening and they are more likely to become confused and upset. The most common reason this happens is that they become tired. Handling the demands of living with dementia may be manageable in the morning when they're fresh, but after a long day of confusion, their ability to cope starts to wane, and they're more likely to become frustrated and engage in problem behaviors.

If you find that your parent experiences sundowning, a good idea is to structure the day so that anything challenging happens in the morning. Ideally doctor's visits and other complex activities can be scheduled as early in the day as possible. Evening activities can be much more simplified and less demanding. Another good strategy can be to encourage your parent to rest or to take a brief nap after lunch so that he or she won't be so tired toward the end of the day.

It can sometimes be helpful to pair an activity that your parent likes with one that your parent doesn't like, so as to make the disliked activity seem like less of a hurdle. If a parent doesn't like getting dressed or undressed, for instance, it might be easier if doing so is associated with a favorite game or music or other activity.

In general structuring the environment and structuring the day provide context. Chapter 12 on communication emphasized the importance of providing context when talking with a parent, but the same is true for the environment—the more parents' surroundings and daily routine become familiar, the more likely it is that they'll be comfortable and not to need to engage in disruptive behaviors.

Many adult children complain that their parents with dementia follow them around incessantly, never leave them alone, or get upset when they leave, even for only a short time. This behavior can in itself sometimes be experienced as problematic. Usually the reason parents latch onto children in this way is that they don't know how to handle the environment and their children provide ongoing clues about how to act and how to navigate things. But if the environment and the routine are structured such that they themselves provide a lot of clues, your parent will be less dependent on your constant presence.

Bathing and Sleeping

Bathing and sleeping are often among the biggest challenges for dementia sufferers and can trigger a lot of problem behaviors.

People with dementia can be highly sensitive to water temperature or can become disoriented when they are in a tub or shower. Resistance to bathing is extremely common, and for many families the inability to bathe a loved one is a key reason they bring in personal-care help or choose a care facility.

It's often helpful to schedule baths early in the day when the parent has more energy and is less confused. Bathing is also an area in which it can be useful to pair something unpleasant with something your parent likes—he or she might be more amenable to bath time if it is accompanied by favorite music, for instance, or favorite snacks, aromatherapy (or favorite perfumes or aftershaves), or a gentle massage. Another approach to encouraging bathing is to make it seem like a preparation for something your parent enjoys. "Your son Bill is coming over this afternoon," you might say. "Let's get ready!"

Sleep problems—including being unable to fall asleep, waking up frequently at night, and frequent daytime napping—are a common issue with dementia because the disease can affect the part of the brain that governs the normal circadian rhythm. In addition some medications that help forestall the memory problems of dementia can have the side effect of disrupting sleep.

Once again structure and repetition can help. A regular bedtime and a regular routine for getting ready for bed can make the transition easier. So can soft music. In order to prevent waking up during the night, you can try to limit fluid intake before bed and encourage your parent to use the bathroom before going to sleep. If your parent does wake up during the night, a night-light can help prevent disorientation and falls.

You might also want to talk to your parent's doctor to see if any sleep problems are being caused by something other than dementia, such as sleep apnea or restless legs syndrome.

Exercise and Activity

Problem behaviors are less likely to occur if a dementia sufferer experiences sufficient stimulation and activity. Not *overstimulation* of course. Too much happening at once is a recipe for trouble. But complete boredom can also lead to frustration.

Apart from its physical advantages, exercise is useful in keeping people with dementia engaged and happy (and tired enough to sleep well).

Many scientific studies have shown that exercise is remarkably effective in reducing agitation and depression among dementia sufferers.

Of course very few older people with dementia can do an elaborate workout, but even simple arm and leg stretches and walks down the hall have a lot of benefits. It's a good idea to have your parent's doctor or a physical therapist who works with the elderly suggest an exercise routine tailored to your parent's abilities and needs. The most important elements are aerobic exercises, such as walking, strength training to improve mobility, and stretching.

Occasional activities can also help parents to feel happy and comfortable. They can include listening to music, playing simple games, reminiscing, looking at picture books or photo albums, knitting, and so on. Anything that stimulates the senses can be valuable. You can make a game of asking your parent to feel different textures or to identify items in a bag by touch (such as a spoon, a comb, or a toothbrush). Painting with watercolors can also be fun. Some family members create a rummage bag full of interesting items that parents can spend time looking through if they get bored.

Often when care partners are busy with a project, such as preparing a meal, parents will ask "Can I help?" Of course the truthful answer might be "no," but this is another case where you want to respond to feelings and not just words. Your parent is very likely asking for an activity. Assigning a parent to do something simple and safe (folding napkins, for instance) can create a feeling of usefulness and satisfaction, as opposed to frustration.

Allow (Some) Choices

Parents with dementia often feel that they have lost all control over their own life. They don't know what's going on, and they don't know how to reassert control. Loss of control is a principal source of frustration and fear. So, anything you can do to create a sense of autonomy on your parent's part is likely to help reduce fear and frustration and thus head off problem behaviors.

Regularly offering your parent choices is a good, easy way to deal with this problem. They don't have to be monumental choices—they can be as simple as orange juice versus apple juice or whether to wear a white shirt or a blue shirt today. But routinely allowing parents to choose one option over another is a way of reassuring them that they still have some say over their own lives.

When offering choices, it's a good idea to limit them to two (or if necessary three) very specific options. Open-ended choices—such as "What kind of juice would you like?" or "What do you want to wear today?"—can actually backfire and provoke anxiety. It's generally better to offer two limited alternatives.

Offering choices is especially useful when engaging in an activity that makes your parent anxious. If you parent is nervous about bathing, questions such as "Do you want to wash your face yourself, or would you like me to help?" can restore a sense of autonomy. Offering choices can occasionally work as a strategy to get parents to do something about which they're reluctant. For instance, parents who don't want to go to bed might be coaxed into bedtime by being asked which nightgown or pajamas they want to wear.

Choices aren't always a good idea—sometimes parents are tired or irritable and don't want to have to expend the mental effort required to make a decision. But very often being able to exercise a choice reduces frustration and fear.

Don't Accuse or Challenge

In general when people are becoming frustrated or afraid, one of the last things they need is for someone to put them on the spot. When challenged, their natural tendency is to lash out.

In taking care of a parent with dementia, it can seem like the most natural thing in the world to ask a question such as "Why did you do that?" or "What were you trying to do?" It can also seem natural to correct your parent and explain that he or she made a mistake. We don't say such things to be mean; we say them because we genuinely want to help.

However, to parents who are already frustrated or afraid because they're not sure what's going on, these kinds of questions can seem like an accusation. Often parents can't answer the question "Why did you do that?" because they don't know, or they can't find the right words. As a result, the question makes them even more frustrated and confused and causes them to feel as though they did something wrong. Similarly explaining that they made a mistake doesn't necessarily help them to understand what happened; it can just make them feel bad and even more frustrated and scared. And this response can make a problem behavior more likely to occur.

It can be incredibly difficult for a care partner to behave in a way that can't be misinterpreted as challenging or accusatory. Nonetheless trying to simply accept whatever happened and sympathize is often the best way to prevent a difficult situation from becoming even worse. This is one more situation where paying attention to feelings, not just words, is a key to success.

Plan Ahead

Finally it's a good idea to plan ahead for how to cope with truly difficult problem behaviors, such as if a parent becomes highly agitated and aggressive. What will you do in such a situation? Is there someone you can call? Can you discuss the possibility with that person ahead of time?

The exact response you choose will depend on a great many factors but, as always, being proactive and planning ahead is better than reacting on the spot. If such a problem occurs, you'll be a lot calmer and more effective if you already have a plan in place than if you have to improvise in the moment.

20

How to Handle Problem Behaviors
When They Occur

When responding to a problem behavior, the goal is simple: Minimize the harm and move on. But just because the goal is simple doesn't mean that it's easily accomplished. It can be very difficult, in part because many types of harm simply can't be minimized. A parent who adamantly refuses to go to a medical appointment creates a lot of practical difficulties for which there is no easy solution. If a parent breaks something valuable or does something highly embarrassing in public, the damage is done and there's no way to undo it.

But minimizing the harm and moving on can also be difficult because care partners are human beings too, and they have natural human reactions.

As a care provider you are, in a sense, in a position of authority. When a parent engages in problem behaviors, it's easy to experience them, at a minimum, as a challenge to your authority. In some cases you might also experience certain behaviors as a direct insult, as insufferable intransigence, as willful stupidity, or as bullying. Even if you don't consciously think of your parent's behaviors in this way, in the split-second when they occur it's virtually impossible not to have a visceral reaction of anger and defensiveness. And that's okay. You're a human being, and these are natural, in-the-moment, involuntary reactions.

The problem though is that if you act on these reactions, it will only escalate the tension and make the situation even worse. Parents with dementia aren't intentionally being brats; they're confused and acting out of fear and frustration. If your parent is then confronted with anger and defensiveness, it will only add to the fear and frustration and perpetuate a vicious cycle.

So what's important in responding to problem behaviors is to (1) accept your own reactions but (2) then act in a contrary way. In fact you often need to literally "act," in the sense of playing a role and behaving somewhat artificially. This isn't easy; it's a skill, but it can be learned over time. The goal is to play at being a calm, wise, reassuring figure who can relieve the fear and frustration, even though you might actually be angry and resentful inside.

If you think about it, this is a technique that parents of toddlers learn as well. Fighting or arguing with a toddler is useless; you just need to minimize the harm and move on. But dealing with a toddler is generally easier because it's obvious to you and to others that a small child doesn't have the capacity for adult reasoning and comprehension and the ability to regulate moods and emotions. With a parent, however, you're used to the person being a fully functioning adult. It's very hard to shrug off difficult behaviors because you can't just tell yourself that the person is only a small child. It takes a lot of effort in the heat of the moment to remember that your parent is not acting intentionally and is suffering from a brain disease.

And if it's hard for you, it's even harder for other people to understand. Everyone instinctively comprehends that toddlers misbehave because they're immature, but because many people go through life with little experience of dementia, they often don't immediately understand why your parent is behaving in a peculiar way. When a toddler has a meltdown and starts throwing a tantrum in a grocery store, few people will be shocked and many parents will immediately sympathize. But when an 80-year-old throws a tantrum in a store or adamantly refuses to be examined in a dentist's office, it's far more distressing and embarrassing.

So here are some tips for responding effectively when your parent starts engaging in problem behaviors.

Pick Your Battles. Remember that a good goal for your relationship is to always ask "What's most important?" In many cases, if you look at a situation with some perspective (which can be difficult to do when you're tired and short-tempered), what seem like problematic behaviors may well be more of a nuisance than something dangerous or harmful. If your parent is spending all afternoon rummaging through drawers or making a mess that's easy to clean up, it might not be worth the effort to try to put a stop to it. If your parent refuses to take a bath one day or refuses to eat lunch one time, it might not be worth arguing over (unless it becomes a consistent pattern).

Thus it's a good idea to ask yourself whether the behavior is simply annoying or is something that will actually cause harm. Of course annoying behavior is unpleasant, but you have to weigh putting up with it against the fact that trying to stop the behavior could result in even more unpleasantness. Sometimes it's best to save your energy for situations where it's truly needed.

Stay Calm . . . or at Least Act Calm. Difficult as it may be, take a deep breath and respond to your parent with exaggerated calmness. Model the behavior you want your parent to exhibit. Your parent may be agitated and anxious, but it's difficult to remain upset for long when the person you're speaking with is sanguine and unflappable.

Staying calm can be very difficult when your parent does something socially embarrassing. Often the best way to deal with such situations is with a sense of humor—an awareness that "today's embarrassment is tomorrow's joke." Of course embarrassing behavior is almost never funny at the time, but it frequently becomes a source of amusement when recounted later, and keeping this fact in mind—seeing how you might tell the story at some future date—can sometimes help. Responding with a sense of humor yourself can also defuse other people's tension and upset caused by your parent's behavior; it signals quickly that your parent "didn't mean it" and is suffering from confusion.

Staying calm is also difficult when your parent insults you or accuses you of wrongdoing. If your father accuses you of stealing his wallet, it's natural (but usually not very helpful) to get offended and deny it. A better response might be "I'm sorry your wallet is missing. I'll help you look for it." If your mother accuses you of mistreating her, it's usually best to simply ignore the direct accusation and listen for feelings, not just words. You might say, "I'm sorry you're feeling mistreated. That must make you feel terrible. Would it help if I did *x*?"

Respect What Your Parent Is Experiencing. If your parent is agitated and upset, it's because whatever he or she is experiencing is agitating and upsetting—however much it might seem like nonsense to you. For this reason, it's usually of little help to tell your parent to calm down or to say that whatever your parent is worried about is not a real problem. These responses are likely to make your parent feel belittled and unheard—and simply increase the level of frustration.

Remember, "if you can't fix it, sympathize." Accept your parent's feelings and experiences, sympathize, but remain calm yourself.

With a toddler, sometimes the solution to a tantrum is simply to give the child a big hug. But touching or hugging people with dementia when they're upset is not necessarily a good idea and can cause an instinctive negative response. Some parents respond by flailing or hitting in this situation. Usually the best way to react to your parent's agitation is to back off and provide more personal space, not less. A good physical response is to stand back at a 45- or 90-degree angle—not face-to-face—with your hands at your sides and your palms open.

Asking "What's wrong?" seems logical but it isn't always a good idea. While the question sounds sympathetic, the problem is that people with dementia often can't articulate exactly what's wrong—which only makes them more frustrated.

You might also be tempted to use logic to prove that what your parent is worried about isn't serious. But people with dementia are unlikely to be able to follow logic, especially when they're agitated to begin with, and they may experience your efforts as once again contradicting what they believe to be real. Remember that you want to respond to feelings, not just words.

The best approach is usually to stay calm and sympathize. Once your parent calms down a little, you might cautiously explain (without directly contradicting what your parent said) why you don't view the issue with as much concern.

Unfortunately sometimes parents will experience your steadfastly remaining calm as itself a form of not taking their concerns seriously. They will then try to goad you into getting upset, just so they can feel that you truly understand how they feel. This is frustrating, but the truth is that if you *do* get upset, it won't make your parent feel any better and it will only make the whole situation harder to resolve. Most parents will eventually capitulate and calm down, although it sometimes takes them quite a while to run out of steam.

Use Distraction. One silver lining with dementia is that people who have it are often easily distracted. Not always; sometimes they get fixated on certain ideas and won't let them go, and people who are upset and agitated are less likely to simply move on to a new topic. But in many cases, memory impairment means that it's harder to stay focused on a particular subject. So when parents start engaging in a problem behavior, it's often a good idea to simply try to distract them.

Sometimes doing so is as easy as changing the subject ("I wonder if the mail has arrived") or asking a simple yes-or-no question ("Would you like some lunch?"). Sometimes you might bring up something else your parent is concerned about or enjoys.

Some people go so far as to create a "distraction kit" that can be used if they need a way to change the subject. This could be a box of interesting items—a music box or sound machine, a photo album, books with interesting pictures, games, simple puzzles, souvenirs, and so on.

Distraction is tricky. If you try to distract parents too abruptly ("Hey, let's look at this book!"), they might experience it as another form of belittling or not taking their concerns seriously. Distraction works best when it seems natural. For instance, you might listen and sympathize with your parent and at the same time start making a snack. After a while you can ask, "Do you want grapes or cheese?" or some other question that seems incidental to the conversation. Gradually you can ask more questions, or ask for help, and redirect your parent's attention.

Another option is to try to turn the subject toward something unrelated that you're concerned about (or can pretend to be). For example, "I'm sorry you're so upset. Actually, I've been upset too lately. I'm having an issue at work. I'd like your advice. Can I tell you what's going on?"

Distraction is usually the only available weapon when your parent's problem behavior involves disinhibition, or engaging in socially embarrassing behaviors. If your parent is undressing in public, insulting people, or using inappropriate language, you can't really just stay calm and sympathize. You need to find some way to distract him or her and head off the problem. In the worst case, you may need to do whatever is necessary to remove your parent from the situation and then do your best to calm things down afterward.

Distraction can be extremely difficult if your parent has reached the point of having a lot of trouble understanding language, although it might be possible to use nonverbal cues.

Use a Checklist of Possible Causes. Once you've dealt with the immediate crisis, it's often a good idea to run through a mental checklist of what might be causing the problem behavior to see if there's some way to minimize it. For instance:

- Is your parent hungry, thirsty, or tired?

- Although it can sometimes be hard to tell, does he or she have pain or physical discomfort?

- Has there been a sudden change in the environment?

- Is your parent overstimulated (such as by an intense TV show)?

- Is the environment too loud? Too busy? Too cluttered?

- Was your parent trying to do something that was too difficult?

- Is your parent experiencing delirium?

When parents start taking off their clothes, this can be a sign that their clothing is too tight, too warm, or otherwise uncomfortable, or that they need to use the bathroom. Wandering can also be an indication that a person needs to use the bathroom.

When problem behaviors suddenly increase in frequency, especially if they involve delusions, the cause might also be a urinary tract infection or other medical condition unrelated to dementia.

In general problem behaviors almost always have some cause or reason. They're not random. Engaging in a difficult behavior is a way in which parents can communicate that they have a problem—and it may well be the only way in which they're able to do so.

Don't Talk about It Afterward. Once the problem behavior has stopped, it's usually best to ignore it and not bring it up later. It's generally impossible to teach your parent that the behavior was a mistake or not to do it again. Bringing it up later only calls your parent's attention to whatever it was that was so upsetting in the first place. This is the second part of "minimize the harm and move on"—once you've minimized the harm and the crisis is over, move along and do your best to forget about it.

21

Responding to Your Other Family Members and Friends

Siblings, other relatives, and friends are often tremendously helpful in taking care of a parent with dementia. They can be extremely generous in offering their time, financial help, and emotional support.

But here's a dirty little secret about dementia care that people don't talk about much: In a lot of cases, the exact opposite is true. Family members can disappear like ghosts when you need time off. Far from offering support, friends may be unable to understand the difficulty of what you're going through or be uncomfortable discussing the subject. Family members may be in denial and unwilling even to acknowledge the problem. Relatives often sharply disagree about what kind of care is appropriate, especially when the costs of caregiving begin to add up. And it's not uncommon for the people who provide most of the care to be accused by other family members of not doing a good job, exaggerating their workload, or even angling to get an unfair share of an inheritance.

In short dealing with the rest of the family can sometimes be almost as much of a struggle as dealing with your parent's illness.

This chapter offers some perspectives on handling relationships with family members when they're not being as supportive as you would like, as well as on talking about the disease with young children and teenagers.

Dementia Is a Family Disease

In some cases of course family members are simply unreliable or irresponsible people in general, and if that's the case, it's probably an issue that you've been dealing with for a long time. But very often, what happens is that fairly healthy family relationships start to become strained and break down because of the pressure brought to bear by the difficulty of a parent's dementia. That's the problem that we discuss here.

Let's face it: Dementia is difficult to deal with for everyone. Many family members don't want to acknowledge what's happening because it's painful or scary. Many people experience grief and don't know how to express it. They don't feel able to make the necessary time or financial commitments but don't want to admit that they can't, so they become defensive. And some become needy or offended because the role they're used to playing in the family has been displaced.

In short *dementia is a family disease*. Everyone in the family is negatively affected in one way or another. And the symptoms of a family disease often express themselves in family disharmony.

Of course, if you're the primary care provider, that's the last thing you need. In order to take care of your parent, you need support, not squabbles. Many care partners are already at the breaking point as a result of the responsibilities they have for their parent, and further family issues are enough to push them over the edge.

What can you do?

A good place to begin is to acknowledge three things:

1. *You need to look after yourself first.* Remember, self-care is not an afterthought. It's the key to being able to perform your role as a care partner. In the same way that you have to prioritize looking after yourself in order to take care of your parent, you have to prioritize looking after yourself over "taking care of" your relatives who are not behaving as they "should." It's often necessary to simply walk away from disagreements with relatives in order to preserve your peace of mind.

2. *You need to look after your parent second.* Although dementia may be a family disease, it's your parent who has the critical symptoms. Taking care of your mother or father in the right way, however difficult it may be, trumps doing something else just because another relative is advocating it.

3. *You can't "fix" your family.* Many people in this situation become consumed by anger and frustration. They feel unappreciated, disrespected, hurt, and used. And that might be entirely accurate—but the truth is that, at the moment, there's nothing you can do about it. Family

members who are behaving in this way are typically doing so because they're in denial, scared, defensive, or feeling hurt themselves. Because your relatives are so motivated, there's no way to logically argue them into understanding how hard you're working or what your needs are. Complaining about their behavior is akin to beating your head against a wall. A better approach is simply to accept your relatives' attitudes for now and then figure out, given your situation, the best way to care for yourself and your parent.

Setting Goals for Your Other New Relationships

When family members are unhelpful, it's often best to apply the same goals to your relationship with them as you're applying to your parent. For instance:

ASK YOURSELF, WHAT'S MOST IMPORTANT?

If your brother or sister isn't shouldering a "fair share" of spending time looking after your parent, this lack of cooperation might be infuriating. But starting an argument isn't likely to solve the problem. Chances are, it will simply make your sibling defensive and even less likely to help.

In this situation, what's most important isn't that your sibling does the work; it's that the work gets done and you're relieved of a crushing burden. Most of the time, it doesn't really matter who does it. Rather than fighting with your sibling, it might be more productive to find a friend who's willing to give you some relief so you can enjoy yourself instead of arguing.

Some people in this situation find that friends are willing to step in and offer help. (Often, it's somewhat unlikely friends who turn out to be the most willing.) A friend might volunteer to spend time playing cards with your parent, knitting, doing puzzles, sharing stories, and so on— particularly if your friend also enjoys those activities. And a friend might also think of other ideas or activities that you wouldn't.

Some caregivers are angry because they feel that it's their sibling's job to relieve their burdens, not their friend's. But what's most important is simply that someone is doing it. For the time being, your friend is filling in and doing the job—and that's totally fine.

LISTEN TO FEELINGS, NOT JUST WORDS

In the pressured environment of a family with dementia, relatives often say things that simply aren't true and are hurtful. It's easy to take offense and become defensive yourself. But this is a situation where it's useful to listen to feelings and not just words.

For instance, sometimes siblings or other relatives resent a child who is the primary care partner. They may accuse the child of exaggerating symptoms, promoting dependence, or seeking undue control over the parent.

In reality the other relatives may be feeling guilty that they aren't contributing more themselves or fear that they will be less loved (or perhaps less remembered in an inheritance). This is a difficult situation. In some cases, such relatives' feelings can be assuaged by involving them more by asking their opinions on a lot of relatively unimportant matters (your parent's favorite foods and activities, for instance). You might not want to elicit their views on topics that are very important to you or that you understand far better than they do, but any way in which you can make them feel involved without causing them a lot of work may be likely to reduce the backbiting by making them feel less guilty and removed.

It's also important to remember that siblings often have different relationships with their parents. Some may be more independent, and others may be more deferential. Some children are unwilling to take away their parent's car keys no matter how dangerous the situation has become. It's good to understand that an ostensibly objective debate about proper caregiving can really be about underlying parent–child emotional relationships.

Different people grieve in different ways too, and some conflict between siblings over caregiving is actually the result of different ways of dealing with grief.

I'LL FIX IT IF I CAN . . .

The goal of "I'll fix it if I can, and if not, I'll sympathize" doesn't fully apply here, because you're unlikely to truly sympathize with unhelpful relatives. However, there may be ways that you can fix things or at least make them a little better.

With relatives who are not shouldering their fair share of the work, one approach is to treat the relationship as a business transaction or a charitable appeal. "I understand you're extremely busy," you might say, "but would you be able to commit to a regular shopping trip on Wednesdays? Would you be able to commit to x dollars a month to help pay for a home health aide? Would you be able to commit to 2 hours every other weekend for yard work and larger projects around the house?"

This approach won't always work, but relatives who are feeling guilty about not doing enough may be willing to make a relatively minor but regular commitment of time or money. Such offers make them feel that they are helping out, and while it might not be nearly as much as you need, at least you'll know what you can expect and what you have to fill in elsewhere.

This approach usually works best if you tailor your request to what you think your family member would be most likely to be willing to do. While it's natural to ask for whatever kind of help you happen to need most at the moment, securing a commitment for any kind of help is better than asking for assistance and getting a noncommittal response.

Another strategy is to document the number of hours you spend taking care of your parent and/or your parent's financial situation. It can be easy for relatives to grossly underestimate how much work you're doing or how expensive providing care is. Providing exact figures can remove an excuse for not helping out.

With relatives who are in denial or who think that you're exaggerating your parent's condition, a solution that sometimes works is to get an authority figure to back up what you've been saying all along. For instance, you might be able to get your parent's doctor to hold a family conference and explain your parent's symptoms, how much care is needed, and what's likely to happen in the future. The doctor might be able to explain that you can't do everything yourself without help. Sometimes relatives are more willing to listen to a third party in a lab coat than to you.

If they are, resist the urge to say "I told you so" or "That's what I've been telling you all along." That may be true, but what's most important is that your family accepts what the doctor has told them, not that they acknowledge that they were wrong. Pointing out that they were wrong is likely to cause them to become defensive and to reject the doctor's opinion. If they want to think that they were right all along and that it's only *now* that your parent's condition is as bad as you've been saying, that's okay. You've still accomplished your goal.

A common dementia phenomenon is that parents will have difficult symptoms around their usual care providers, but when they're around a stranger or someone they don't see that often, they will suddenly get "better" and their symptoms will seem much less severe. This is often called *showtiming*, because it's as though the parent is suddenly on stage and has to perform. It can be very frustrating for regular care partners because relatives who only occasionally drop by will see the parent at his or her best and not understand what the care partner's burden is like most of the time.

A doctor who deals regularly with dementia might be able to explain the showtiming phenomenon at a family meaning, and indicate that for this reason other relatives might not have a good grasp of the parent's general condition. This explanation might help relatives to acknowledge that they were "wrong" about how bad things are because they can say that it wasn't their fault.

THE "GOOD ENOUGH" RELATIONSHIP

This chapter discusses dealing with friends and relatives who aren't very helpful to you, but it's important to acknowledge the other side of the coin—as you spend more time taking care of your parent, you might be less available to be a good friend or sibling to others who might need you.

While it's important to take care of yourself, and that includes maintaining healthy friendships, it's also important to acknowledge that some of those friendships might become a bit less close for a while as you're consumed by caring for your parent. That's okay. You don't have to maintain perfect relationships during this difficult time; you only have to maintain "good enough" relationships.

So that no one feels slighted, it can be a good idea to explain at the outset to people you care about what you're going through and how it will get worse. Some people write a letter or a social media post to explain the situation to all their friends and more distant relatives. Such a message can point out the progressive nature of the disease and apologize in advance if you're not able to be as close or responsive as you have been in the past. Another advantage of this kind of message is that it might prompt offers of help. If it does, accept them!

RESPECT YOUR OWN BOUNDARIES

Much of this chapter discusses walking away from unproductive conflicts with family members. This is a form of respecting your own boundaries.

Another situation that can challenge your boundaries occurs when another family member *is* deeply involved in a parent's care or is otherwise upset by the situation, and comes to you looking for support. This need for sympathy is reasonable in general of course but sometimes what happens is that family members try to offload all of their stress onto you—which is the last thing you need given all the stress you're already under. (This is not uncommon when a dementia sufferer's spouse is involved in the care, but it can happen with other relatives as well.)

Respecting your own boundaries is important here too. It's fine to be a sympathetic listener, but at the point where family members are in effect asking you to function as a therapist, you might want to gently suggest that they find an actual therapist or at least join a support group where other people in addition to you can listen and provide encouragement.

On a different note, walking away from unproductive emotional conflicts with family members doesn't mean that you should stop listening to your relatives' views altogether. An irony of the situation is that family members who *aren't* deeply involved in day-to-day care—even if frustratingly so—occasionally have ideas or perspectives that can actually be valuable. Sometimes their distance gives them an ability to perceive changes over time that are hard to notice if you're with your parent every day. They sometimes are better able to see the "big picture" or to think outside the box and come up with new ideas. You might be upset that they're not more helpful in the everyday tasks of providing care, but that doesn't mean that you can't occasionally take advantage of their ideas if they would in fact be helpful to you or to your parent.

Dealing with Children

Dealing with family members who are young children or teenagers is another issue altogether. Children tend to experience the same reactions to dementia that other family members do: stress, guilt, anxiety, and so on. But they're usually less able to understand and communicate their feelings. As a result, it's important to talk openly with them and help them to cope—difficult as this inevitably is when you're simultaneously trying to take care of your parent.

When a grandparent develops dementia, younger children often react with fear. This fear can be caused by a wide variety of issues, such as the inability to communicate with the grandparent, the grandparent's unpredictable behavior, the possibility that the grandparent will become agitated and upset, or the grandparent's inability to express love and affection (or perhaps even recognize the child). Some children are afraid that the disease is contagious and that they might get it. Others can't understand what causes the illness and are afraid that it's somehow their fault.

For this reason, it's a good idea to explain to children as best you can that dementia is a brain disease, that you can't "catch" it, that it's not their fault, and that their grandparent doesn't love them any less even though he or she might no longer be able to express it very well. As always, the best way to counter fear is with information, although you might have to tailor the information to the child's age level.

Teenagers are usually able to understand that a grandparent has a disease, but their reactions can still be complicated. For instance, it's common for teenagers to resent a grandparent who has dementia and who is causing them to have to do extra work, absorbing all their parents' attention, embarrassing them in front of their friends, or making it impossible to engage in normal family activities. On a subtler level, teenagers might feel frustration that there's no way to "fix" the situation or enable the grandparent to get better.

There's no easy solution to this problem, but it's generally good to allow teenagers to talk openly about their feelings. Telling them that it's wrong to be angry about a grandparent is usually unproductive because they will typically just get more frustrated or else repress their feelings and then express them in some other way. Grandparents with dementia *are* frustrating, and denying this fact helps no one. It's fine to let teenagers talk about how they feel and even to share your own frustrations. The goal should be to encourage an attitude of "loving the person but hating the disease."

Many teenagers are embarrassed to talk to their friends about having a grandparent with dementia, but it's often a good idea to encourage them to do so. It can give them an opportunity to vent and might make them feel less awkward about inviting friends to their home if their grandparent will be there. They might also discover that a number of their friends are in the same position, in which case they might bond and form what is in effect a miniature support group.

IV

The Later Stages

22

Moving Your Parent to a Care Facility

Some relatives manage to care for a person with dementia at home for the entire course of the disease. This choice can in a sense be a heroic act, because the demands on a care provider are usually overwhelming as dementia reaches its later stages. Most of the time though, as dementia becomes advanced, it ceases to be either wise or even possible to care for the person at home. At some point it's likely to be necessary to consider moving the person to a care facility.

It's important to recognize that moving your parent to a care facility is *not* a failure on your part, or a sign of giving up, or a betrayal of your parent's wishes. Some people view a move to a care facility as one or all of these things, but this is simply not true.

It's not a failure. Some care partners assume that it's their responsibility to care for a dementia sufferer at home no matter how difficult it becomes. The problem with this attitude is that it doesn't accept the reality that dementia is not just the natural course of getting older; it's a complicated, debilitating brain disease. While many aspects of early dementia care can be handled at home by a family member, at some point it becomes better and healthier for the person with the disease to be cared for in a specialized facility.

The irony is that many people who think they should take care of their parent at home wouldn't even contemplate avoiding specialized care in this way if their parent had a different type of illness, such as cancer or lung disease. With such illnesses, we naturally assume that seniors will fare better in a hospital or other specialized care environment where they can be looked after 24 hours a day by trained staff members. The myth that a caregiver should look after a dementia sufferer at home no matter what is really just a result of the myth that dementia is a normal age-related decline, not a tragic and difficult disease. Once you truly understand that dementia is a disease, it becomes easier to accept that people in the advanced stages need to be cared for in a specialized environment.

It's not giving up. Another myth is that moving your parent to a care facility somehow involves giving up hope or assuming that your parent's life is over. This is not true. Of course because the disease is progressive and incurable, family members can't really hope that it will just go away. But the point of moving parents to a care facility is not to give up on them; it's to allow them to be in an environment where they will be safe and will have the best chance for a good quality of life, because they will receive intensive, round-the-clock support and care of a sort that a single care partner or family couldn't possibly be expected to provide.

Parents with dementia need a lot of care for their physical as well as their emotional needs. No one can be on call to satisfy both at all times. Moving a parent to a care facility allows you to share the physical demands with others, and frees up your energy to attend to higher-level emotional needs. Far from giving up on your parent, it's a way to increase the amount of care and love that your parent receives.

You should also note that your parent won't be confined permanently to the facility. You can still take him or her out for walks or medical appointments or to visit your home or go to a restaurant—although you might find that doing so is at times difficult and disorienting for your parent.

It's not a betrayal of your parent's wishes. At some point, many parents who are starting to decline with dementia will beg their children not to "put me into one of those places." (They might also have said something similar earlier in life in connection with taking care of their own aging parents.) As a result of this attitude, it can be wrenching for children to contemplate moving their parents, and making this decision can make children feel very guilty.

It's important to think about what parents actually mean by such statements, and it's especially important in this context to listen to feelings and not just words. When parents ask not to be "put away," they're expressing fear. They're scared of a disease that is robbing them of their faculties, and they're especially scared at the idea of being abandoned. They're saying to their children in effect, "Please don't abandon me." The thought of "one of those places" has come to stand in for the idea of being abandoned and left someplace where they will have no control and no idea about what's happening to them.

So it's important to keep in mind that moving your parent to a facility that can provide a more appropriate level of care is very different from abandonment. You're not betraying your parent's wishes because you will still be there to care for emotional and other needs.

That's not to say that parents aren't initially scared and disoriented when they move into a facility. They typically are, at least at first. However, imagine that your parent could magically not have dementia for just a moment and you could ask, "Do you want to remain in a place where your needs can't be cared for, where you can't be kept safe, and where your family is being crushed by overwhelming burdens?" Almost certainly you'd find that your parent would prefer not to be in such a situation.

Types of Care Facilities

Some people are surprised to discover that there is a wide range of facilities geared to older adults. They include:

Retirement communities are housing developments limited to residents over a certain age, such as 50 or 55. They don't typically have special care for dementia or other disabilities, but they usually offer group activities of common interest to older people.

Assisted-living facilities are communities for older people (and occasionally younger people with disabilities) who want additional help with activities of daily life. Independent residents typically live in apartments where they have no maintenance worries and often have access to prepared meals in a common dining area. Assisted-living residents may get an hour or two a day of additional help from a staff member with cleaning, dressing, bathing, and so on.

Memory-care facilities are specialized communities for people with dementia. Typically they are staffed round-the-clock with aides and are locked so that residents can't wander outside unattended. Meals, housekeeping, and some nursing care are provided. Residents often live in small apartments—sometimes with a roommate—and most of their time is spent in common areas where there are often social and other activities. Sometimes a memory-care facility is a separate unit within a larger assisted-living facility.

Nursing homes are acute facilities for people who need round-the-clock skilled nursing care. Some nursing homes have a separate area within the facility for residents with dementia.

Continuing care retirement communities, or CCRCs, are facilities that combine most or all of these features in one residential campus. People often move into them while they can still live independently or need assisted living, with the understanding that if they later need memory care or a nursing home, they can be transitioned to a higher level of care without having to leave the community.

Advantages of a Memory-Care Facility

Although many people focus on the downsides of memory-care facilities, it's important to remember that they can also have a lot of advantages. Some of the potential advantages include the following:

Help with Physical Care. No matter how dedicated family members are, it's impossible to provide the same level of physical care as a full-time staff. This is especially true in situations that require heavy lifting.

You Can Focus on Higher-Level Needs. Because other people are taking care of your parent's physical needs, meals, and so on, you can focus on spending quality time with your parent. You can laugh, reminisce, and respond to your parent's emotional needs with more attention. This is a big advantage.

Social Interaction. Most memory-care facilities encourage residents to join in a variety of social activities. This sort of interaction with peers can be very helpful to seniors with dementia—and it's very hard to provide it if you're taking care of a parent on your own.

Mental Stimulation. A lot of memory-care facilities provide activities for mental stimulation, including live music, painting or drawing, crafts, and games. They may also provide opportunities for physical exercise. You could provide these activities on your own of course, but it's extraordinarily difficult when you're also taking care of someone's physical needs, and it's very hard to arrange for live music and group activities of the sort that many facilities offer.

Relief for You. It can be a tremendous relief to know that your parent is being looked after around the clock and you don't have to worry at all hours about safety. It can also be a tremendous relief to have some time for yourself. Remember, self-care is nothing to feel guilty about. It's an important part of being able to care effectively for another person.

A STRUCTURED ENVIRONMENT

In addition to the other advantages offered by memory-care facilities, one of their most underrated benefits is that they provide a highly structured environment.

Most memory-care facilities operate on a routine. Meals are served at the same time each day, and residents often wake up and go to bed at the same time. Activities are tightly organized and often occur on a repeating schedule. The environment is carefully planned to be pleasant, soothing, and not disruptive. Residents are encouraged to spend time in common areas and activities rather than by themselves. Residents' rooms are typically much smaller and simpler than assisted-living apartments— in fact they can often resemble dorm rooms.

The goal of this very structured setting is to help residents remain calm, reassured, and oriented. The core experience of dementia is not knowing what's going on in the environment. By making the environment as simple and as routine as possible, it's easier for residents to orient themselves to what's happening and not to feel lost at sea.

Interestingly one of the reasons that people so often react negatively to the idea of "being put in one of those places" is that it seems to represent a loss of autonomy. For most healthy people, the idea of living in a small room, of following the exact same schedule every day, and of not having a lot of privacy is very depressing. The prospect seems boring and unpleasant. But it's worth remembering that people with moderate or severe dementia experience the situation very differently. For them, having a large home and unscheduled time can seem scary and disorienting. Having an easy-to-navigate environment and a clear schedule can make them feel much more reassured.

When Is It Time?

There's no one clear right time for your parent to move to a care facility. It all depends on your unique situation. However, in general family members should consider such a facility when it becomes clear that a parent's needs have begun to exceed what the family can reasonably provide.

It might be time to move a parent to a care facility if:

- A family can no longer keep the dementia sufferer safe. For instance, if a parent is getting up and wandering outside at 3:00 A.M., this behavior may be more than a family can be expected to handle. The same is true if a parent is experiencing frequent episodes of agitation and aggression.

- Care providers become so drained that their emotional or physical health begins to suffer, or they are unable to keep up with work and other responsibilities.

- The physical demands of caring for a dementia sufferer (such as lifting or moving the person) become too difficult to handle.

- The dementia sufferer becomes incontinent on a regular basis. For many families, the difficulty of cleaning up after incontinence—and the perceived indignity to a dementia sufferer of having this task handled by a family member—are the "last straws" that prompt a transfer to a facility.

Many families put off a move to a care facility as long as possible, and delaying the move can be a noble effort. However, it's often the case that dementia sufferers who move to a facility earlier—when they have more of their faculties intact—experience a better long-term positive adjustment than those who move after the disease has progressed to a more severe stage. Moving later, when a parent is more confused in general, can be more disruptive and upsetting.

Many family members say that they know that their loved one will eventually need to move to a facility but that the loved one "isn't ready yet." The truth is that, in a very large number of cases, it's the family member and not the loved one who isn't ready. The person with dementia has often been ready for some time to move to a place that offers more intensive care.

The problem with saying that a loved one "isn't ready yet" is that it's usually left unclear what would constitute being "ready." In practice it's sometimes a bad fall, a scary wandering incident, or some other event involving serious potential or actual harm that finally persuades the family member that additional help is needed. But a parent with dementia shouldn't have to risk the possibility of a serious injury in order to be ready to move to a place that can provide more appropriate care.

A move to a facility is always a disruption in a parent's life and will almost always generate complaints and a temporary worsening of symptoms. They are to be expected. It doesn't mean that the move was a mistake, and it doesn't mean that it would have been better to wait—since waiting could cause the temporary worsening of symptoms to be even more extreme.

Respite Programs

Some assisted-living and dementia-care facilities offer *respite* programs, which allow a senior to move to the facility on a short-term basis, such as for a few weeks or a month, without a permanent commitment. The idea is that they offer a respite or vacation for the senior—although the reality is that they offer a vacation for the care partner. The programs can be good and can give a care provider a much-needed break. They can also be a way of determining how well a senior adapts to a residential program.

There are some cautions that should be noted though. One is that it's common for care partners to opt for a respite program at a point where they're at their wits' end. The break is helpful, but afterward the parent comes home, and the care partner goes right back to being extremely stressed. If the care partner is truly at the breaking point, it's probably a sign that the parent needs to be in a facility on a more permanent basis. Moving a parent back and forth from a facility to home again can be more stressful and disruptive for everyone involved than simply permanently moving the parent to a facility.

A second caution involves sending parents for a brief stay at a facility to "try it out" and "see how they do." The problem is that a move to a facility is disorienting by its very nature and almost always results in a temporary worsening of symptoms. Thus a family member might conclude prematurely that the parent isn't doing well, especially if the family member communicates to the parent (directly or indirectly) that the arrangement isn't necessarily permanent, which makes the parent less willing to commit to the environment and the routine.

Making a Successful Transition

There's no way to guarantee a smooth transition to a dementia-care facility, but there are steps you can take to make the move go as smoothly as possible.

It's not necessary to give your parent a lot of advance notice about the move. Your parent likely won't remember the discussion, and it might cause unnecessary anxiety or even resentment.

On the other hand, some families take the parent to visit the facility ahead of time, perhaps for an activity or a meal. You don't have to say what the facility is or that you plan to move your parent there; you can just say that you're going to visit some people. But ideally your parent will be less bewildered by the surroundings because they won't be completely unfamiliar.

It can be good to ask the facility staff for advice on making the transition easier. The staff members will have handled this situation many times and probably have a very good sense of what works best.

Even though you might be fretful or nervous, it's good to act as positive as you can. You can explain that your parent is lucky to be able to stay in such a wonderful environment with caring people. You can describe all the activities to look forward to. And you can reassure your parent that you will still visit regularly.

It's not necessary to insist to your parent that the new arrangement is permanent. You might feel more comfortable saying something vague, such as that it's "for now," which is not really a lie since it *is*, at a minimum, for now. It's not at all uncommon for new residents in a memory-care facility to tell everyone they see that they're only there for a day or two. This is a self-comforting mechanism. Accepting parents' reality and allowing them to believe that the arrangement is temporary (at least on the day of arrival) can help make the transition smoother. You probably don't want to directly lie and say that it *is* only for a day or two, since that might cause your parent to distrust you and be more resistant to adapting to the environment, but it's okay to be vague and to allow your parent to engage in self-comforting behavior.

Personal belongings can be very comforting to anyone in a new environment. Bringing small sentimental items from home to your parent's room can ease the transition. Such items can also spark conversations with staff members and help to break the ice. Another option is to bring some of your parent's favorite music and ask the staff to play it in your parent's room. Photographs are also good—although you'll want to make sure you have copies of old photos in case they become damaged.

Apart from taking sentimental items, it's best not to overpack. Too many belongings or clothing choices can overwhelm someone with dementia. If you find that you didn't pack something your parent truly needs, you can always bring it later. Also, you'll want to label everything you can with your parent's name—clothes, towels, canes, walkers, and so on. It's very easy for personal items to get lost because other residents can become confused and walk off with them.

If your parent tends to be better at certain times of the day, such as in the morning, it's a good idea to schedule the move for that time. (But check with the staff; in some facilities early morning is a busy time and might not be ideal.)

If possible, talk to staff members ahead of time about your parent's background, hobbies, preferences, and so on. The more the staff members know about your parent, the easier the transition will be.

One of the best times to transition parents to a care facility is if they are already in another facility. For instance, if your parent is in the hospital briefly due to a fall, it can be very easy to move directly from the hospital to a care facility. You can simply say that your parent is going to leave the hospital to spend some time at a place for rehabilitation and continued recovery.

Once your parent has moved to the facility, it can be good idea to visit frequently at the beginning as a form of reassurance that you're still part of your parent's life. However, it may be better to give parents a chance to adjust on their own—to get used to the routine, make friends, and so on. While you might want to take your parent on an outing, it's usually best to wait until he or she has fully adjusted to the new routine before disrupting it with a special trip. (Staff members might be able to give you a good sense of how quickly your parent is adjusting.)

Be prepared for a lot of complaints and unhappiness. It's common for parents to call their adult children frequently to ask where they are or demand to be taken home and to repeatedly pack up their belongings in an effort to leave. Parents might also claim that they're being mistreated and try to make their children feel guilty about the move. You don't want to totally discount specific accusations of course, but many parents will complain about the facility or the staff simply as a way of expressing frustration with the reality of their condition. As always you want to focus on feelings, not just words.

In such a situation, it's usually best not to try to argue or reason with your parent, but to simply express empathy regarding the situation. Remember that a good goal is to say "I'll fix what I can, and as for what I can't, I'll sympathize."

Your Own Feelings

Many caregivers become so wrapped up in worrying about how a parent will feel about moving to a care facility that they neglect to think about their own feelings.

Moving your parent to a care facility is a major transition for your parent, but it's a major transition for you too. It's a good idea to find a close friend or therapist to talk to about what you're experiencing. Many children feel guilty about the move even though they know rationally that it's for the best. Others worry that their parent won't receive perfect care. And ironically many worry that their parent *will* receive great care—that the staff will do a better job than they did and that they will feel inadequate as a result.

Many care partners become so wrapped up in the "job" over time that they actually experience a psychic loss when they no longer have to look after their parent around the clock. It's as though they have lost their raison d'être, and they suddenly have to look for a new identity or work to replace their old one.

Some care partners become dismayed as a result of other people's reactions. Friends or family members may view your decision to move your parent to a care facility as a failure or as a selfish choice. Of course this reaction is usually ridiculous. Friends and relatives might mean well, but unless they have actually taken care of someone with dementia, they have no idea what the responsibility involves.

The next chapters discuss how to choose a facility, how to pay for it, and how to relate to parents once they have moved into one.

23

How to Choose a Care Facility

Choosing a dementia-care facility for your parent isn't easy. As with everything else in the world of dementia, it's a good idea to plan ahead. If possible, visit several facilities before you think your parent is ready for one. These visits allow you to become familiar with what these facilities do, so that you can feel more comfortable with the transition when the time comes. It will also give you a better sense of when your parent has reached the point where a care facility is appropriate.

Touring several facilities can help you decide which one is best for your parent. Knowing in advance where you want your parent to go might not seem essential, but the truth is that many older people end up needing full-time residential care as a result of a crisis or a sudden downward spiral. Trying to make a difficult choice about where to send your parent when you have a lot else on your mind in such a situation can be very difficult, and you'll be very happy to have investigated the possibilities ahead of time. Another consideration is that many facilities have a waiting list. Putting your parent on a waiting list early can ensure that a space will become available later when you need it.

If you think that a facility that you visit might be a good candidate, you can ask for references. It's always helpful to speak with other family members who have a loved one there and who can share their experiences.

If you make more than one visit to a facility, do so at different times of the day so that you can get a fuller sense of the operation. But if you're comparing two facilities, you might want to schedule your visits to them for the same time of day. Many people with dementia experience sundowning and become more agitated and disoriented as the day goes on. Thus if you visit one facility in the morning and another in the late afternoon, you might get a skewed sense of how comparatively happy and alert the residents are.

What to Look For

Communities for people with dementia generally fall into two categories, depending on whether the resident has serious medical problems *other* than dementia that require significant or round-the-clock care. Residents who have no significant problems other than dementia are usually cared for in an assisted-living-type environment. This is a social model of care in which residents are provided meals, housekeeping services, activities, companionship, and other benefits.

People who have other serious medical problems might require a nursing home, sometimes called a skilled nursing facility, that is equipped and licensed to provide medical services.

In the United States, nursing homes are heavily regulated by the federal government. In response to widespread reports of nursing home abuses, Congress passed a law in 1987 that required nursing homes to comply with a wide variety of federal requirements in order to qualify for reimbursement from Medicare and Medicaid. Some states have adopted their own nursing home requirements in addition to the federal ones.

Assisted-living-type facilities generally don't qualify for Medicare or Medicaid though; as a result very few federal requirements apply to them, and they are regulated almost entirely by the states. The states vary a great deal in how stringently they monitor facilities and in what services these facilities are allowed to provide. For instance, some states severely limit the ability of employees to administer medications and offer other routine health-related services. Many family members are surprised to discover what types of services employees can and can't perform. State agencies' websites often provide information on this topic, and it's helpful to become at least generally familiar with what kinds of services you can expect; you can find more information in the Resources at the back of the book.

In terms of what to look for in a care facility, this chapter focuses mainly on assisted-living-type arrangements, although many of the same considerations apply to nursing homes as well.

There are three major criteria to keep in mind when comparing care facilities. One, you want a place that will meet your parent's physical needs—provide a safe environment, healthy food, adequate medical care, assistance with daily life activities, and so on. Two, you want a place that will meet your parent's emotional needs—where you think your parent will be happy, or at least as happy as possible. This is a place where the staff members are kind and responsive and there are opportunities for social and recreational activities. And three, you want a place that your parent can afford.

There's an old saying among business vendors: "You can have it good, fast, or cheap—pick two." Ideally you'll be able to find a care facility that perfectly meets all three of the criteria described in the previous paragraph. However, in some cases you might need to compromise and figure out which combination of features best meets your needs if you can't find one place that is perfect in all respects.

Meeting Physical Needs

In terms of meeting your parent's physical needs, a good first question is what sorts of medical care are available. Does the facility have a doctor, a nurse practitioner, or a registered nurse on site? If not, is such a person on call? What about nights and weekends? Be aware that some assisted-living-type facilities have only a "wellness nurse," who can perform routine checkups but can't respond to serious medical problems.

If your parent has a medical issue that the available staff can't handle, what is the procedure? Will they call you? Will they have your parent transported by ambulance to an emergency room? Also does the facility have transportation available for routine medical appointments? How is dental care managed?

If your parent needs physical, occupational, or speech therapy, or needs a private aide, does the facility provide these services, or does it regularly coordinate with outside providers? Do the staff members routinely communicate with outside providers to ensure that important information isn't missed?

It's important to ask what the facility's policy is for dealing with behavioral issues, such as wandering and aggressiveness. Are residents ever restrained? What does the facility do if a resident develops truly difficult behavioral issues? Are antipsychotic medications ever used? Does the facility have a relationship with a behavioral health clinician who can make recommendations and coordinate care between the facility and the resident's doctors?

Another important question to ask is the resident-to-staff ratio. For the best care, you'll want a ratio of no more than six to one; five to one is better. Be sure to ask what the ratio is at night and on weekends. Most facilities will have fewer staff members on duty at night, but keep in mind that dementia can cause people to be awake at night and need care. Do the staff members routinely check in on residents at night? If so, how often? Do they wake them? Many facilities also have reduced staff on weekends, but if the staff is reduced too much, it can leave residents feeling abandoned and needing attention. You'll also want to ask what sorts of specialized training are given to the staff regarding dementia care.

Quality meals are important, and you'll ideally want to visit during mealtime to get a sense of whether the food is healthy and appetizing. Do the residents have a personalized nutrition plan? Can the kitchen accommodate people who are diabetic and others with special dietary needs? Can it provide kosher meals? Will the staff provide feeding assistance if it becomes necessary?

How does the facility handle mobility problems? Will it give you statistics on how often residents experience falls, and does it have a program in place to reduce falling? Can the facility accommodate residents who need two people to lift them?

Does the space strike you as a safe and secure environment? Is it easy to navigate? Do residents have room to move around, have access to the outdoors, and get regular exercise? A lot of research has been done lately on how lighting, floor surfaces, paint colors, signage, and so on can help dementia sufferers to stay oriented. Have any of these principles been incorporated into the facility's design?

What is the facility's attitude toward family members? Are families encouraged to participate in care plans and communicate directly with staff members? How are families kept informed about changes in a resident's condition or needs? Does the facility sponsor family gatherings and support groups?

What level of personal-care assistance is provided? Is the facility able to provide additional levels of care as your parent's needs change? How is incontinence managed? Can the facility accommodate residents who are bedridden or limited to a wheelchair? Does it offer hospice care or have a relationship with an off-site hospice provider?

Questions about housekeeping and laundry services and about

whether a podiatrist and a hairdresser or barber regularly come to the site are also appropriate.

In the United States, if you live close to a state line, you should be aware that different states have different rules for care facilities, which might affect whether you want your parent in one state or in a different one. In some states, for instance, a care facility nurse can administer injections, apply creams and ointments, give someone eyedrops, draw blood samples, or cut residents' pills in half for them, but in other states doing these tasks may be illegal. And states can have different rules about whether a facility is required to honor a "do not transport" provision in a living will.

A Happy Environment

In addition to making sure that your parent's physical needs are met, you'll want to find a place that will take care of emotional needs.

By far the most important factor in this regard is the attitude of the staff to the residents. You can pick up on this by talking to the staff members and observing how they interact with the people who live in the facility. Is there a pessimistic attitude that nothing can be done, or an optimistic feeling that much can be done to make the residents happier and more comfortable? Are difficult behaviors treated hopelessly as a sign of brain damage or as a sign of unmet needs that can be investigated and addressed?

These factors are intangible ones that can't be answered with statistics, but they're critical to knowing how comfortable your parent (and you) will be with the facility.

One statistic you *can* inquire about, however, is staff turnover. How long do staff members who look after residents typically work at the facility after they've been hired? Low staff turnover tells you that the people who work there like their jobs and feel well treated and supported. High turnover can be a red flag for bad management or poor conditions; it's especially a problem in a dementia unit because it means that residents frequently have to get used to new people, which is difficult. In general residents do better when they have stable relationships with staff members who come to know them well.

Another way of addressing the attitude of the staff is to ask how flexible the arrangements are. Is personal care provided on a strict schedule, or does the timing sometimes depend on the resident's needs? Is there a set list of activities, or are the activities sometimes shaped by what the residents seem to enjoy most? Asking this question is another way of inquiring how much individual attention the residents receive. This factor can't be overstated. If the residents feel loved and cared for, that's far more important than whether socks sometimes go missing or the food is occasionally bland.

As for activities, ask what they typically include: music, exercise, games, pet visits? Is there much variety? If the dementia unit is part of a larger assisted-living facility, are there occasional joint events, such as concerts? Are there activities scheduled in the evenings and on weekends? You might want to check the activities schedule and observe whether an activity that is scheduled during your visit is actually taking place—some facilities provide visitors with a wonderful list of activities that is seldom followed in practice.

You can learn a lot about a facility by observing the residents and the physical setting. Do they seem relaxed and comfortable? Are they well-groomed, clean, and dressed? Does the facility group residents by cognitive level? Does the facility include residents who have psychiatric diagnoses other than dementia? Does the environment strike you as clean and neat? Are there a lot of distractions (and potential sources of overstimulation) such as clutter, paging announcements, or blaring TVs?

Other questions include: Are the rooms private, or will your parent have a roommate? Is it okay to bring a lot of sentimental items? Are there specific visiting hours (and if so, do they work for you)? Is it generally okay to visit during meals? Is there access to religious services?

Another question is whether there is a specific person on staff whose job it is to communicate with families about how residents are faring and how their needs might be changing. If so, how often does this communication typically occur?

Financial Questions

The last of the three criteria is whether your parent can afford the care facility.

In order to make this decision, you'll need to fully understand the cost structure. For instance, some facilities have a simple monthly fee, while others (especially those where the dementia unit is part of a larger assisted-living community) may have a base charge for rent and a separate charge for care. Some retirement communities require you to buy an apartment for a large upfront cost, which you can then sell back to the community when your parent leaves or passes away, usually at a discount that becomes larger the longer your parent lives there. Such communities may have a monthly fee as well.

Even if the facility has a simple monthly fee, you'll want to make sure you understand what the fee includes. Will you be paying separately for regular extra services, such as haircuts, nail care, podiatrist visits, laundry, and transportation? What about supplies, such as adult diapers, bathroom tissue, cleaning products, and so on? Will you be expected to provide these items, or will the facility provide them—and if it does, will there be a separate charge for them?

You'll want to ask about the facility's discharge policy. Does it ask residents to leave if they become disruptive, require a higher level of care than it can provide, experience multiple falls, or run out of money? If the facility is capable of providing a higher level of care, how will this factor affect the fee? Will the fee go up, and if so, how much? If your parent runs out of money, will the facility accept Medicaid?

Be aware that some facilities may require you to provide proof that your parent can pay for care for a minimum amount of time, which may be several years.

Again the physical, emotional, and financial aspects amount to a three-legged stool. Making the stool balance can be very difficult, and at least some trade-offs are almost always necessary.

24

How Am I Going to Pay for All This?

The idea of paying for a full-time dementia-care facility for an indeterminate amount of time is overwhelming to many families, especially those who are not so rich that they can easily write a check for round-the-clock care and not so poor that they can easily qualify for government benefits. This chapter looks at a number of options for such individuals that are available in the United States. (Some suggestions for other countries appear in the Resources section.)

The first thing you should know is, if you're worried about paying for care, you're not alone. The second thing is that unfortunately there might not be a lot of help available—and what help *is* available is often hard to access, and you might need to consult a lawyer or financial planner.

As with everything else involving dementia, planning ahead and looking into what financial assistance is available early can pay big dividends.

The chief problem for families is that the health care and health insurance systems are focused on *medical care*, defined as professional services that can be provided only by a person with advanced skills and training, such as a doctor or nurse. Medical care is different from *custodial care*, which is helping people who need assistance with activities of daily living, such as meal preparation, bathing, dressing, or using the bathroom, or who need constant supervision to keep them from falling or doing something dangerous.

Our system is set up to help people access medical care, not custodial care. In one way this makes sense, because if older people start to need help preparing meals, we don't usually think of that as a health care issue. But in the case of dementia, it *is* a health care issue—the reason a dementia sufferer needs help is because of a *disease*, and the difficulty is a symptom of the disease. Just as families often make the mistake of not treating dementia as a real disease, so our health care and insurance systems also tend not to treat it as a real disease and not to provide help to the people who have it.

Another issue is that the health care system is often willing to pay only for *treatments*, meaning interventions that will prevent an illness, cure it, or make it better. For people with dementia, custodial care does not involve treatment, although it greatly improves their quality of life. This lack of coverage is another example of the system being prejudiced against people with dementia: It's not their fault that science hasn't come up with an effective treatment for their disease, and it seems like a scandal that it's so hard to get dementia sufferers the care they need just because the medical system doesn't yet have a solution for it.

However, this is the sad reality that so many families face. This chapter provides a look at the landscape of paying for dementia-care facilities.

Private Insurance and Medicare

Most private health insurance plans cover doctor's visits, inpatient hospital care, and prescription drugs. They might also cover nursing home care if it's necessary for a medical reason, that is, if the person has a medical condition that requires skilled nursing. But these plans typically won't cover custodial care even if it's necessary because of dementia.

Medicare, the federal government's insurance plan for the elderly, is much the same in terms of coverage. In many cases Medicare will cover up to 100 days of nursing home care (with a co-pay after the first 20 days) as long as there is a "skillable need," meaning that the person needs medical treatment and not just help with activities of daily living. But purely custodial care isn't covered.

Medicare typically covers nursing home care only if the person has first been in the hospital for 3 days. And the person must have been admitted to the hospital for those 3 days. Be careful: Sometimes a person will be in the hospital for several days "under observation," but won't technically be admitted. If nursing home care afterward is a possibility, you'll want to consult with your doctor about whether your parent has officially been admitted.

You might be able to avoid the 3-day rule if your doctor participates in something called a "Medicare Accountable Care Organization Shared Savings Program."

Many people buy Medicare supplemental insurance policies, often called "Medigap" policies, to cover whatever Medicare doesn't, such as co-pays. Unfortunately, these policies typically won't cover custodial care.

Long-Term Care Insurance

A growing number of people are buying long-term care insurance to cover custodial care in old age. Of course by the time a parent is developing dementia, it's probably too late to buy a long-term care policy at a reasonable cost. But if your parent purchased long-term care insurance a while ago, the policy might be extremely beneficial.

However, you'll want to get a copy of the policy and look carefully at what's covered. There is no standard policy; every company is different, and there are a lot of variations. For instance:

- Many policies say that coverage kicks in only if the person is unable to perform certain activities of daily living without help, such as dressing, bathing, or using the bathroom. Activities of daily living are often referred to as ADLs. Different policies have different lists of ADLs, and some say that the person must have difficulty with a minimum number of ADLs—one or two might not be enough. You might also need to have a doctor or other professional certify that your parent needs help with certain ADLs.

- Some policies don't provide any coverage until a person has been at a facility for a certain length of time, such as 30 days.

- Some policies pay for only a portion of the facility's cost, and there is usually a maximum amount that the policy will cover over your parent's lifetime.

- Some policies will pay for long-term care at a facility, but not for room and board. This is an enormous loophole, inasmuch as housing and meals account for a large part of the cost of a facility. Some facilities charge separately for room and board, but many don't and simply have an all-inclusive fee. In the latter case you might need to ask the facility to try to break down the costs.

Social Security

Social Security is best known as a retirement program that people pay into while they're working, but the agency also separately provides Supplemental Security Income to needy seniors and disabled people to bring their income up to a certain level. Furthermore, almost all states offer an "optional state supplement" in addition to the federal SSI payment.

Happily this optional supplement can often be used to pay for assisted-living care. The supplement is typically paid directly to the facility.

Unfortunately the amount of the state benefit is unlikely to pay the full bill. In most states it ranges from a pittance to a few hundred dollars a month; the most generous states offer around $1,000. And these amounts are income dependent, so even parents who qualify for the program might not qualify for the full monthly benefit.

Medicaid

Medicaid is a joint federal–state program designed to provide health care to the needy. Each state operates its own version of the program, and the rules vary considerably from state to state.

The good news is that, at least in some cases, Medicaid will pay for custodial care, but generally only if the care is provided in a nursing home. This often creates the anomaly that Medicaid covers care in a memory-care unit if the unit is part of a nursing home, but it wouldn't cover the exact same memory-care unit if it were part of an assisted-living facility.

The bad news is that it can be very difficult to qualify for Medicaid. The program is designed for the truly needy, and there are very strict asset and income qualifications. In terms of assets, a person has to be virtually destitute to be eligible. In terms of income, even Social Security and a small pension can be enough to disqualify a recipient.

Some people try to sign up for Medicaid by giving away a lot of their assets, but the government can disqualify you for a period of time if you have given away assets during the last few years (known as the *lookback period*), so this typically doesn't work.

In most states, the lookback period is 5 years from the date you apply for Medicaid. If you gave away assets during that period, the state will add up the amount you gave away and divide it by the average monthly cost of nursing home care in the area; the result is the number of months that you'll be ineligible for benefits after you otherwise qualify.

In 2021 the *penalty divisor* (that is, the average monthly cost of nursing home care) was about $7,000 in Ohio and about $14,000 on Long Island in New York. So if you gave away $14,000 during the lookback period, Medicaid wouldn't cover you for the first month after you qualified on Long Island or the first 2 months after you qualified in Ohio.

If you owned a house worth $350,000 and you gave it to someone, you'd be ineligible for more than 2 years on Long Island and more than 4 years in Ohio.

In practical terms, the effect of the Medicaid lookback rules is that many people have to spend down their assets paying for long-term care and then, when they finally run out of money, they can receive Medicaid.

If your parent is married, there are special rules that allow people to qualify for Medicaid while their spouses can retain enough resources to provide for themselves. But these rules are complex and vary by state.

There are some other exceptions. An important one is the Caregiver Child Exception, which allows a parent to transfer ownership of a house to a child without a lookback penalty if the child lived with the parent in the house for at least 2 years, the child provided care for the parent during that time, and the parent would otherwise have had to be in a long-term care facility. There is also an exception for certain gifts to benefit a child who is disabled.

Applying for Medicaid is tricky. Because of the lookback period, you might have to account not only for your parent's present finances, but also for old bank accounts and other financial assets from a number of years ago. And of course your parent likely has no memory of what happened to these assets.

You'll also have to account for gifts made by your parent that include not just major donations, but even checks written in connection with a birthday or wedding.

In general planning and applying for Medicaid is incredibly complicated. While there are a few people who have successfully navigated it on their own, it's almost always necessary to consult an elder law attorney or a financial planner with a specialty in Medicaid to avoid falling into the many traps for the unwary.

MEDICAID WAIVERS

While it's generally true that Medicaid pays for a nursing home but not assisted living, there are some exceptions. A key one is that nearly all states have adopted Home and Community-Based Services waivers (sometimes called 1915(c) waivers) that allow them to pay for services outside a nursing home in certain situations. Many of these waiver programs benefit seniors with dementia.

The goal of these programs is to allow seniors to avoid a nursing home for as long as possible by paying for services that will allow them to live at home or in an assisted-living facility, as long as the costs involved are no more than they would be in a nursing home.

Under these programs, Medicaid won't pay for room and board in an assisted-living facility but, depending on the state, it might pay for nursing care, personal care, housekeeping, transportation, social and recreational activities, case management, medication management, and personal emergency-response systems.

Of course this still leaves the conundrum of how a person poor enough to qualify for Medicaid can afford to pay room and board in assisted living. Some states limit the amount that assisted-living facilities can charge once a resident qualifies for Medicaid. And some facilities voluntarily offer discounted rates for a small number of Medicaid-eligible residents. Also many states allow seniors who qualify for care under a waiver program to keep more assets than they would be allowed to under standard Medicaid policy.

Other Options

If your parent is a veteran, it's worth contacting the Veterans Affairs (VA) office in your area about possible benefits. The VA typically doesn't pay for full-time memory-care facilities, but it sometimes provides benefits greater than those offered by Medicare, including adult day centers, respite care, and resources specifically geared to caregivers.

Two other options for seniors to raise cash deserve mention, if only because they are widely touted in advertisements: selling life insurance policies and reverse mortgages.

SELLING LIFE INSURANCE

There's a growing industry that will buy life insurance policies, typically for more than the cash surrender value but less than the value of the death benefit. The owner of the policy gets a lump sum, and the buyer takes over paying the premiums and collects the full benefit when the person dies.

This transaction is often called a life settlement, although if the person has a terminal illness and a life expectancy of less than 2 years, it's often referred to as a viatical settlement. A viatical settlement is more likely to be tax free than a life settlement. The result of such a settlement is a quick infusion of cash, but the family also loses the expected benefit of the policy.

If you're trying to qualify your parent for Medicaid, you should know that the cash surrender value of a life insurance policy is typically counted as an asset when determining if you qualify. If you sell the policy, it's no longer an asset, but the amount you receive for it will be considered an asset. You might have to spend all the money on long-term care before qualifying for Medicaid, so you won't necessarily come out ahead.

REVERSE MORTGAGES

Like a regular mortgage, a reverse mortgage is a loan that's secured by your home. The difference is that, with a reverse mortgage, you don't have to make monthly payments to the lender. Rather the entire amount of the loan comes due when you die, sell the home, or move.

Some people use reverse mortgages to access their home equity without having to sell their home or make monthly loan payments. It's a bit like selling your home but still being able to live there.

Reverse mortgages are available to people age 62 and older. The proceeds of the loan can be taken as a lump sum, a monthly annuity, or a line of credit. The owner is still responsible for property taxes, insurance, utilities, and so on.

Such mortgages might help some people, but they're not necessarily a good choice for parents planning on long-term care for dementia because, once parents move into a long-term care facility, the entire loan will become due. (An exception is if your parent moves into a facility but your parent's spouse is a co-borrower and continues to live in the home.) There are also high closing costs for such loans that are typically rolled into the loan but which you'll never get back.

One problem with both reverse mortgages and selling life insurance is that they can pit generations against each other (and sometimes pit siblings against one another) by cashing out an expected inheritance. They also can create unexpected tax issues as well as problems qualifying for Medicaid. It's always best to talk to an elder law attorney, estate planner, or specialized financial planner before undertaking such a significant transaction.

25

Your Relationship with Your Parent in a Care Facility

Once your parent moves to a residential dementia-care facility, your relationship with your parent will change—so it's good to give some thought ahead of time to how to make the most of it.

For many people, the most significant change they experience is that *they're no longer in charge*. They may have been used to organizing their parent's life, making all the major and everyday decisions about their care, and having the last word. All of a sudden, that's no longer the case. The facility is providing round-the-clock staffing and is in charge of your parent's day-to-day activities, meals, and personal care. The facility is now your parent's home. Your interaction is reduced to being a visitor on someone else's turf.

To a lot of family members, this is a disturbing development. While the respite is obviously welcome, they also feel, in a sense, displaced. And they worry—they worry that the facility isn't taking proper care of their parent, that the meals and activities aren't all they should be, and that the staff aren't caring for them the way they would or the way they imagine that their parent would want to be cared for.

Of course if you want to find fault with a care facility, it's easy to do so. Most residents are unhappy at first about the transition and may express their feelings by criticizing their living conditions or care, so it's easy to build on a parent's complaints. And dementia care is, by its very nature, imperfect. The symptoms of the disease are such that there will be constant unscheduled needs for the staff to attend to, with the result that personal items may get lost and activities may not happen exactly as planned.

However, if you express an overall sense of dissatisfaction with the facility's handling of your parent's care, this isn't necessarily helpful to your parent. Your parent needs to feel at home and comfortable in the new surroundings, and will take a lot of cues from you—so if you convey happiness with the environment, your parent will be much more likely to be soothed and relaxed.

It's important to remember that a move to a care facility is a significant transition for both you *and* your parent. It's not just your parent who is experiencing a big change in lifestyle. It can be very hard for a caregiver to "let go" and allow other people to care for their parent, especially when they aren't family members, and they necessarily handle caregiving differently because they're managing an entire group of residents with different levels of functioning.

So it's important to step back and remember why your parent is in the facility. Your parent is there because of needs that can no longer be met at home. The purpose of the facility is to provide for those needs. The positive side is that, because the facility is now providing for those needs, you're now freed up to attend to more important, higher-level needs—needs for familial companionship and emotional support that a paid staff can't provide—and that you likely weren't able to provide very well previously because you were overwhelmed dealing with more basic physical requirements.

Relating to the Staff

As a family member, relating to the staff at a dementia-care facility is very important. It's much more important than in other types of institutions, because staff members play a much larger role in your parent's life than they would in an assisted-living retirement community, for instance, and they will take care of your parent for a much more extended period of time than they would in a hospital.

It's wise to have a constructive relationship with the staff. That's not to say that you shouldn't complain occasionally if staff members are doing something obviously wrong, but it's good to be understanding of the pressures that the staff are under in dealing not just with your parent but with other residents who might have very different needs. If you want something done differently, it's good if possible to couch your idea as a suggestion in the spirit of working together to meet your parent's needs, rather than as a complaint.

Because dementia care is so difficult, it helps to keep your expectations reasonable. Personal items will get lost. The staff will ignore your parent occasionally when they have to attend to an emergency involving another resident, just as they will sometimes ignore other residents when your parent has an emergency.

Remember too that the staff members who care for your parent on a regular, day-to-day basis have a job and that your parent and the other residents are the job. You're not. It's very easy for the staff to come to see family members as extraneous, because family members are usually there for relatively short periods of time and because staff members typically receive a lot of training on how to take care of people with dementia but unfortunately often get zero training on how to relate to family members.

A good question to ask staff members is "What can I do to help you?" You might find out that your parent is running low on shampoo, or now needs adult diapers, or is complaining about not having enough blankets. You also might find out about minor health issues or about personal-care problems that you can easily address. Keeping open lines of communication will help everyone to take care of your parent better. You will generally get the best results if you can create the sense that you are working with the staff as part of a team.

Occasionally the staff might inform you that your parent had a minor fall, became agitated and tried to leave the facility, or engaged in inappropriate or embarrassing conduct. It's easy to become alarmed by these reports (or even to look for someone to blame). But it's important to recognize that these behaviors are completely typical for someone who has dementia. The best approach is usually to express concern and ask how you can work together with the staff to minimize the problem in the future.

Some family members go out of their way to "humanize" their parent for the staff. One daughter created a display on her mother's door that included old photos of her as well as descriptions of her job and education, hobbies, likes and dislikes, and so on. Doing so ensured that the staff members who interacted with her mother got to know the person her mother was before she developed dementia.

In general a good attitude is to let the staff take care of your parent's physical needs and to focus on taking care of your parent's emotional needs. This is a good time to hug your parent, express love, and be reassuring about the environment. Although your parent's disease may be advanced, you may find that you draw emotionally closer at this time because you can focus exclusively on your emotional bond.

If you truly have a problem with a staff member, it's wise to raise it with the facility's management, ideally approaching the matter with a problem-solving attitude. One issue that sometimes arises, for instance, is that a staff member will call and ask the family to resolve a behavioral issue or handle some other problem that would appear to be the facility's responsibility. In this case, speak to management and try to get on the same page as to what's expected if the problem arises again in the future.

Visiting Your Parent

Visiting a parent in a dementia-care facility can be very difficult, in part because you often don't know what to expect. Will your parent recognize you? Be happy to see you? Be asleep? Be angry and complain that you haven't been to visit in 3 years—even though you were there just the previous day? It's common for family members to steel themselves before they walk in because they have no idea what they'll find.

In practice, where possible, it's a good idea to pause for a few minutes beforehand and breathe deeply or engage in other relaxation techniques. Parents with dementia will follow your cues, and if you appear stressed, they may pick up on this fact and feel more stressed themselves.

Also keep in mind the tendency of adult children to project their own feelings onto their parents. Many adult children, for instance, feel sad and guilty about their decision to move their parents into a facility. As a result, when they visit they exude a sense of unhappiness or guilt about the fact that the parents are where they are, and they unconsciously assume that the parents feel something similar. And this is true even if the parents in fact feel well cared for and comfortable in their surroundings. You might not be able to help being sad yourself, but it's a good idea to try to avoid communicating this feeling to your parent and not to simply assume that your parent feels the same way that you do.

Many people don't know what to talk about during a visit. Not only will your parent probably be unable to carry on a detailed conversation, but you may find that many of the topics that normally function as small talk don't work very well. For instance, if you ask what your parent has been doing since your last visit, it's likely that your parent won't remember—and may be embarrassed by this fact. On the other hand, you might be reluctant to talk about what *you* have been doing since your last visit, because you might be afraid that such talk will make your parent feel bad about not being able to be at home or to join you.

One way to deal with this conversation gap is to plan to visit during a meal or other activity. In this way you'll be able to engage in doing something together. It may be very entertaining for your parent to engage in music, games, or crafts along with you.

On the other hand, you should be aware that the conversation gap is typically far more awkward for family members than it is for parents themselves. Most of the time it really doesn't matter much what you talk about—the important thing is that your parent knows that you came and that you care. Hugs and laughter mean a lot more than words.

Since people with dementia often tend to lose their short-term memories before their long-term ones, reminiscence is often a good conversational topic. You can say, "Remember that time when . . ." and talk about it. Of course, your parent might not remember the time you're referring to, but if you enjoy talking about it, it's likely that your parent will enjoy hearing about it. And it's possible that your parent will remember, at least after a while. You can generally bring up favorite memories over and over again, because your parent is unlikely to remember that you talked about them on your previous visits.

Other options include singing songs together. Songs often evoke happy feelings and improve people's moods. And even people with advanced dementia are sometimes able to remember song lyrics. You might be able to sing along to music on a cell phone. You can also bring a photograph album or other sentimental object from home and use it to trigger reminiscences.

If the weather is nice and your parent can manage it, taking a short walk or just sitting outside can be a great idea. Fresh air and exercise are healthy, and you can talk about the weather. Being outside often triggers a lot of memories.

Some people with an artistic bent like to create seasonal displays to put in their parents' room to help keep them oriented to the time of year.

It's not uncommon during visits for parents to say, "I want to go home" or to insist on being taken home. Hearing this comment can be very difficult, especially because it can trigger guilt feelings on your part about the fact that you're not caring for your parent at home. Telling parents "You *are* home" is unlikely to be very helpful, and making excuses or promising to take them home another time can simply make them press the issue later.

A good response is to listen to feelings, not just words, and to recognize that the desire to go "home" often indicates a feeling of uneasiness or discomfort. Your parent may be feeling confused or anxious or be experiencing pain or need to go to the bathroom. Gently asking questions to figure out what's prompting this desire and responding to that need can be very useful.

Sometimes another good response is to start a conversation about the person's former home, especially a childhood home. This can trigger pleasant memories and serve as a distraction.

Frequent and Short

As a general rule, frequent, shorter visits are better than occasional, longer ones. Of course, if your parent lives a long distance away, frequent visits might be impossible. But in general, a half hour every other day is better than 2 hours on the weekend. Frequent visits create a sense of continuity and can reassure parents that you're a consistent presence in their lives. You'll also get a better sense of how your parent is faring and any needs that should be addressed. If your visits occur less often—even if you stay for a long time at each one—your observations will be limited to your parent's condition on that particular day. If your parent is having an especially good or bad day when you arrive, you might walk away with a misleading sense of the overall picture. Also frequent visits allow you to interact with more staff members and hear different perspectives on how well your parent is faring.

Another advantage of frequent visits is that it's easier to limit their duration. Visiting a parent with dementia can be very tiring, and if you can keep your visits on the shorter side, it may be much easier for you. It can also enable you to engage in the visits with more energy and enthusiasm. In addition the same may well be true for your parent. Older people with dementia can get exhausted very easily, especially when they have to concentrate on something such as talking with a family member. Some dementia sufferers become noticeably less focused and more irritable after a long visit, simply because they're tired.

Regardless of the length of your visit, a key point is to seem *unhurried*. It's generally a bad idea to approach the visit with an air of being rushed, which is likely to cause your parent to become worried and agitated. If possible, give your parent your full attention for however long you're there. You might want to turn off your cell phone, because a cell phone ringing—even if you don't answer it—can worry or agitate a person with dementia and distract from your interaction.

Even if you can only stay for 10 minutes, it's usually a good strategy to act like you have all the time in the world. If you were visiting a friend, of course, you'd want to start off by saying "I can only stay for 10 minutes," because otherwise an abrupt departure would seem rude. But with a person with dementia, it's very different. Saying "I can only stay for 10 minutes" might make your parent worried and anxious, because it sounds as though something is wrong. You could end up spending the entire 10 minutes just calming your parent down. And while you might worry that a quick departure will seem rude, it's good to remember that people with dementia have an impaired sense of time. Ten minutes might seem to them like 4 hours or vice versa. Many people have spent an entire afternoon visiting a parent with dementia and, when they get ready to leave, their parent exclaims, "But you just got here!"

As a result, the best strategy is usually to simply be present to your parent for as long as you plan to stay and then simply say that you have to go.

A corollary to the "frequent and short" rule is that, given a choice, four separate visits by different family members is better than a single visit by four family members. While you might think that a parent would be delighted to have a visit from an entire family, the truth is that such visits can be exhausting and overwhelming. It's hard for a person with dementia to keep track of everything, and the possibility of forgetting someone's name or identity can be frightening or embarrassing. Short individual visits are generally much easier to handle and allow for deeper interactions than a group get-together.

Of course, family gatherings might make sense on special occasions, such as Christmas or a parent's birthday, but in general they put far more intellectual demands on a parent than short individual drop-ins.

Ending a Visit

Ending a visit at a dementia-care facility can be an art in itself. Parents are often reluctant (and sometimes anxious) about their child leaving.

It's usually impossible for them to pick up on any of the normal subtle cues that people use to indicate that a visit is winding down. On top of this, people with dementia often have no sense of time and very little understanding that the person they're talking with has other obligations that need attention.

However, there are a few techniques that can help. One is to avoid saying, "I'm going to go home." Going home doesn't sound like a pressing obligation, and it can also be a reminder that your parent used to have a home outside the facility. Saying, "I'm going to go home" not infrequently prompts the response "I'll go with you" or "I'm going to go home too."

A better approach is to say, "I have to go do x now." It really doesn't much matter what x is or whether it's truly an immediate need; the point is to convey to your parent that (1) there's a reason you have to leave and (2) it's not your choice. "But I'll be back again very soon," you can add reassuringly.

You can also take advantage of any transition to make leaving easier. If a meal is starting, you can say, "It looks like it's time for you to have some lunch, so I'll see you again soon." The same is true if there's a group activity or even if someone comes in to give your parent medications or if your parent has to go to the bathroom.

Staff members can be very helpful in this situation, since they often understand that ending a visit is difficult. If you can find an excuse to get a staff member's attention, you can tell the person out loud how much you've been enjoying your visit but that you need to go do x now. The staff member might respond by encouraging your parent to say good-bye or by engaging in a distraction long enough for you to make a departure.

If ending a visit is frequently or inordinately difficult, you might plan ahead with a staff member for help in arranging a getaway.

Taking Your Parent Home for a Visit

Sometimes families want to take parents home for a brief visit, such as on Thanksgiving or Christmas. Such visits can be a very nice-sounding idea, but they often don't go as well as expected.

Home visits are often championed by well-intentioned relatives who don't realize how much work is involved in looking after someone with advanced dementia. They might not realize that the three steps in the entryway are now a major obstacle, that your parent can't walk alone without help (and might try to do so and fall, which means constant monitoring will be necessary), or that a family member will have to accompany your parent to the bathroom.

Relatives might also not realize that "home" to your parent is no longer home. Because of the loss of memory, the former home will now to a great extent be a brand new environment, full of difficult expectations and sensory overload. Your parent may become overwhelmed and start exhibiting problem behaviors.

And while your relatives might think that your parent will be disappointed to miss out on a major holiday, the truth is more likely that your parent will have little understanding of the holiday and not be disappointed at all.

Such home visits are often based far more on your relatives' needs and desires than on what's best for your parent. It can be hard to explain this point to your relatives, but hopefully they will begin to understand that visiting your parent in his or her new home at a care facility is generally the better idea.

26

Dealing with the End of Life

While dementia often develops slowly over many years, it is nonetheless ultimately a fatal disease, and it's important to be prepared for this fact, both emotionally and practically.

Because it's a gradual disorder and because most people don't get dementia until they're already elderly, a lot of people who have dementia die from something else. Yet dementia is still responsible for a great many people's passing away. Alzheimer's disease is the sixth most common cause of death in the United States, according to the Centers for Disease Control and Prevention. And the problem is getting worse: Between 2000 and 2018, the number of people dying from Alzheimer's disease increased by 146 percent—while the number of people dying from heart disease decreased by about 8 percent.

And even these numbers are probably low. Cause-of-death statistics are typically based on causes reported on death certificates, but many people are never formally diagnosed with dementia, and others have their cause of death listed as a dementia-related condition such as aspiration pneumonia rather than dementia per se. The result is that dementia-related deaths are probably grossly undercounted.

One study in the journal *Alzheimer's and Dementia* suggested that dementia-related deaths are several times higher than the official count. And a separate study in the journal *Neurology* suggested that for people 75 and older, the real figure for Alzheimer's disease might be five to six times higher than what is reported—which would make it the third leading cause of death for this group, after heart disease and cancer.

Although the symptoms of dementia are highly variable, certain problems often indicate that a person is reaching the terminal stage of the disease. Among them are difficulty in swallowing (or a tendency to choke on foods), being unable to walk or sit upright without help, incontinence, and a near-complete inability to speak.

In the final weeks and days, dementia sufferers often spend a great deal of time asleep or drifting in and out of consciousness, and have shallow breathing or appear to stop breathing for short periods. Their hands and feet (or entire arms and legs) might feel cold to the touch, and they may lose interest in eating and drinking. Because people in this condition can't communicate, it's often difficult to tell if they're in pain. Some signs that a parent might be in pain include restlessness, moaning, sweating, grimacing, and inability to sleep.

Two important concepts at this stage are *palliative care* and *hospice*.

Palliative care is a type of treatment for people with a serious illness that is often provided by an interdisciplinary team of doctors, nurses, and others. Its primary goal is to relieve pain and make the person more comfortable. Palliative care isn't limited to people with a terminal illness, and sometimes people have a palliative care team trying to reduce their pain while a separate medical team is trying to cure them and get them well. However, palliative care often comes into play when a person does have a terminal disease, and the goal of treatment shifts from trying to make the person healthier to simply relieving their pain and discomfort as they continue to decline.

Hospice is a special kind of care given to people with a terminal disease (which includes very advanced dementia). Typically to qualify for hospice, a doctor must determine that there is a greater than 50 percent chance that the person will live less than 6 months.

Hospice is an American phenomenon; outside the United States, the general term is *palliative care*, and the word *hospice* usually refers to a facility that specializes in this type of care. But understanding the distinction is important in the United States, because Medicare doesn't always cover palliative care, but it does cover hospice. Many Medicaid and private insurance plans also cover hospice services.

How Hospice Works

As with palliative care, hospice services are provided by an interdisciplinary team. However, once a person is shifted to hospice care, the medical goal is simply to make the person as comfortable as possible while the incurable illness runs its course.

Hospice services can be provided in a hospital, nursing home, or assisted-living or memory-care facility, but they can also be provided in the person's home. For parents who are not already living in a care facility, choosing to have hospice at home can be very comforting and allow them to pass away in familiar surroundings, rather than in a medical setting. One recent study found that more than 55 percent of hospice care was provided in a home environment.

The hospice team typically includes doctors, nurses, social workers, chaplains, and sometimes volunteers. Palliative care—minimizing the person's pain—is obviously one element, but there are many others. The team works not only with the patient, but also with family members, providing physical, emotional, and spiritual support and sometimes respite care so that family members can get a break. The team coordinates medications as well as medical equipment and supplies (such as providing a hospital bed if necessary). Usually there are regular visits, and someone is available round-the-clock by phone. Someone on the team is usually well versed in ethical concerns regarding end-of-life care.

Some people are resistant to hospice because they interpret it as meaning that they have given up on the person or that death is imminent. This isn't the best understanding. Hospice involves a recognition that the disease of dementia is terminal, but it's not "giving up"; it's simply shifting the nature of the treatment so as to give your parent the best possible quality of life at this stage of the illness. Hospice also doesn't mean that your parent is at death's door; it's simply a response to the statistical likelihood that death may come within a matter of months. Regardless of statistics, some people live longer than expected. The humorist Art Buchwald went into a hospice program expecting to live another 2 or 3 weeks; instead he lived another year and wrote a book about the experience before he died. In fact one scientific study showed that patients who received hospice care lived longer than similar patients who didn't.

Because of family members' fears that hospice equals giving up, many people with dementia don't start hospice care as soon as they could. This is a shame, because the kind of treatment it involves can be extremely comforting to people with advanced dementia (and to their families as well).

One problem in obtaining hospice services is that it can be a lot harder to predict life expectancy with dementia than with other diseases, such as cancer. One survey of hospice providers found that this uncertainty is the leading reason why hospice services are underutilized for dementia patients. It may be necessary to have a detailed talk with your doctor—or to obtain a second opinion—if you believe that your parent would benefit from hospice care.

It should be emphasized that the 6-month criterion doesn't mean that hospice care is limited to 6 months. It simply means that hospice is available to people if a doctor determines that *most* people in the person's condition would be expected to live 6 months or less. Hospice can be provided indefinitely, as long as the person continues to meet this condition.

Grieving the Loss

Losing a parent is always difficult. Losing a parent to dementia isn't just difficult; it's also *complicated*. Many people in this situation don't have the "normal" feelings that grieving children are supposed to have. This can make the experience awkward and unsettling.

A lot of people who lose parents to dementia after taking care of them for a long time don't experience much in the way of grief, loss, or sadness, which may cause them (or others) to question how much they loved the parent. But there's actually a very good reason why their experience is different.

When people lose a loved one suddenly, there's often a period of shock or trauma. When people lose a loved one after a serious illness, there's usually less shock because the death is not unexpected, but there's typically a deep sense of loss and mourning. When a parent dies of dementia, however, you might have much less of a feeling of loss because in a sense the parent you knew and loved hasn't been there for quite some time. You "lost" your parent gradually, over a period of years. You mourned every small loss during that period, every time another piece of cognition or personality disappeared because of the disease. By the end, almost nothing remained of the person whom you loved and remembered.

In other words, you might not feel a sudden onrushing of grief because you've been feeling grief, in small doses, over the entire course of the illness. What you may feel is *relief*. While you're in the midst of taking care of a person with dementia, it's hard to realize how much the ongoing care takes over your whole life. When that burden is lifted, you might feel an odd sense of freedom. You might also feel relief simply because you know how much your parent has suffered, and you know that this suffering is at an end.

Some people also feel a sense of displacement. For a long time, their entire life revolved around being a care partner, and suddenly the entire organization of their life has lost its focus.

Feeling relief instead of grief can make you feel guilty. After all your parent died, and you may think that you're *supposed* to feel a certain way. But there is never a right way to grieve, and certainly there is no right way to grieve a loss as complicated as one from dementia.

After your parent passes away, you'll probably spend a lot of time contacting friends and relatives and telling them the news. This process can also be complicated. Friends and relatives will often feel a distinct sense of mourning and loss, and perhaps even surprise. They haven't been on the journey with you, and they haven't grieved every small loss along the way in the same way that you have. Their reaction can make you feel even more guilty, because more distant relatives and acquaintances are having the very reaction that you think you're supposed to be having. You might even spend a lot of time comforting them in their grief—when, in the ordinary course of events, they would more appropriately be comforting you in yours.

This is very sad. But it's the nature of the disease, which over time slowly robs our loved ones of everything that made them who they were.

In the end though it's not how you react to people's death that matters; it's how you reacted to them all through their life. It's how you cared for them. It's how you asked what was most important, how you listened to their feelings and not just their words, how you fixed what you could and sympathized when you couldn't, how you strove to have a good enough relationship, despite all the losses along the way, and how you took care of yourself so that you could take care of them.

Caring for your parent in this way doesn't just make you a proficient care partner. It is what it truly means to love someone.

Resources

Here is a list of resources for families of people with dementia, arranged alphabetically by topic. Within each topic, resources in the United States are listed first, followed by resources in other English-speaking countries. Programs, websites, and phone numbers are of course subject to change, but every effort has been made to keep this section as current as possible.

Please note that this section is not an endorsement or recommendation of any private company. Also while many of these resources feature lists of service providers, local providers change frequently, and you shouldn't assume that these lists are exhaustive.

ADULT DAY CARE

- You can find local adult day care centers by going to *www.communityresourcefinder.org.* Click on "Care at Home," then "Adult Day Care," and enter your zip code.

- You can also search for adult day care centers on the U.S. Administration on Aging website at *www.eldercare.acl.gov/Public/Resources/Factsheets/Adult_Day_Care.aspx.*

- In the United Kingdom, you can find day care resources at *www.alzheimers.org.uk/find-support-near-you.* For day care centers offered by Age UK, see *www.ageuk.org.uk/services/in-your-area/day-centres.*

ASSISTED-LIVING AND DEMENTIA-CARE FACILITIES

- You can find local facilities that provide dementia care at *www.communityresourcefinder.org.* Click on "Housing Options," select "Assisted Living," then enter your zip code and click "Search." When you get the results, in the left column called "Adjust your search," scroll down to option 4 and select "Provides Memory Care." Then scroll all the way to the bottom of the page and click "Search Again."

- A state-by-state guide to rules and regulations for assisted-living facilities can be found at *www.ahcancal.org/Assisted-Living/Policy/Documents/2019_reg_review.pdf*. You can also find comparative overviews at *www.ncbi.nlm.nih.gov/pmc/articles/PMC4542835* and at *www.aspe.hhs.gov/sites/default/files/migrated_legacy_files/73501/15alcom.pdf*.

- A state-by-state guide to dementia training requirements for different types of care facilities can be found at *www.justiceinaging.org/wp-content/uploads/2015/08/Training-to-serve-people-with-dementia-Alz2FINAL.pdf*.

- A state-by-state guide to dementia training requirements for different types of health care and personal-care workers can be found at *www.justiceinaging.org/wp-content/uploads/2015/08/Training-to-serve-people-with-dementia-Alz3_FINAL.pdf*.

- Medicaid covers assisted-living facilities (to varying degrees) in 44 states and the District of Columbia. You can find a state-by-state guide to this coverage at *www.payingforseniorcare.com/medicaid-waivers/assisted-living#State_by_State_Guide_to_Medicaid_Coverage_for_Assisted_Living_Benefits*.

- In the United Kingdom, the Care Quality Commission offers comparative reports on care homes at *www.cqc.org.uk*.

- In Ireland, you can find dementia-care facilities at *www.alzheimer.ie/wp-content/uploads/2018/11/SCU.pdf*.

CARE MANAGERS

- You can search for local geriatric care managers at *www.communityresourcefinder.org*. Click on "Care at Home," then "Geriatric Care Managers," and enter your zip code.

- There is a professional association for geriatric care managers called the Aging Life Care Association. You can find local members of this group by going to *www.aginglifecare.org* and clicking on "Find an Aging Life Care Expert."

DIAGNOSIS

- You can find local diagnostic clinics by going to *www. communityresourcefinder.org.* Click on "Medical Services," then "Diagnostic Center," and enter your zip code.

- The Alzheimer's Foundation of America offers a free 10- to 15-minute online memory screening test. It's not a substitute for a doctor-administered test, but it may be useful in confirming that someone is having memory difficulties. You can learn more at *https://alzfdn.org/about-afas-national-memory-screening-program.*

DOCTORS

- You can find geriatric psychiatrists by going to the website of the American Association for Geriatric Psychiatry at *www.aagponline.org* and clicking on "Find a Geriatric Psychiatrist." (The search engine doesn't return "nearby" areas, so if you enter your city or town and get no results, try just entering your state and look for someone in your general region.)

- You can also find geriatric psychiatrists by going to *www. communityresourcefinder.org.* Click on "Medical Services," then "Geriatric Psychiatrists," and enter your zip code.

- A U.S. government website allows you to find geriatric psychiatrists in your area and compare them based on criteria such as education and hospital affiliation. Go to *www.medicare.gov/care-compare*, enter your location, and choose "Doctors & clinicians." Click on the "Name & Keyword" box, select "Browse all specialties," and choose "Geriatric psychiatry." Once you see the results, you can click on the "Compare" button next to all the ones that interest you, then click "Compare" at the upper right. (If searching for your specific city or town doesn't yield many results, try searching for your state.)

- You can find some resources for handling dental care for a person with dementia at *www.emergencydentistsusa.com/alzheimers-dental-care.*

EDUCATIONAL PROGRAMS

- The Alzheimer's Association offers live and recorded educational programs about dementia. Go to *www.alz.org* and click on "Your Chapter" to select your area, then click the link for programs.

- The Alzheimer's Foundation of America offers a variety of educational webinars on dementia caregiving at *www.alzfdn.org/webinar_archive.*

ELDER SERVICES AGENCIES

- You can find agencies in your area that provide services to seniors by going to *www.communityresourcefinder.org.* Click on "Community Services," then "Area Agency on Aging," and enter your zip code.
- You can also search for local agencies on the U.S. Administration on Aging website at *www.eldercare.acl.gov/Public/Resources/Index.aspx.* Enter your zip code and click "Search."

FINANCES

- "Daily money managers" are people who help seniors with disabilities to pay bills and handle other day-to-day financial responsibilities. There is a professional organization called the American Association of Daily Money Managers. You can find members near you at *https://secure.aadmm.com/find-a-dmm.*
- In the United Kingdom, you can find a financial advisor who specializes in helping the elderly through the website of the Society of Later Life Advisers at *www.societyoflaterlifeadvisers.co.uk/find-an-adviser.*

GOVERNMENT BENEFITS

- You can find information on Medicare, Medicaid, and veterans' programs in your state by going to *www.caregiver.org/connecting-caregivers/services-by-state,* selecting your state, and clicking on "Government Health Disability Programs."
- Detailed information on Medicare coverage of nursing home care can be found at *www.medicare.gov/Pubs/pdf/10153-Medicare-Skilled-Nursing-Facility-Care.pdf.*
- For information on Medicaid programs in your state that pay for home care services and home health care, go to *www.caregiver.org/connecting-caregivers/services-by-state,* select your state, and click on "Caregiver Compensation."
- For a state-by-state guide to Medicaid waiver programs for dementia care in assisted-living facilities, see *www.dementiacarecentral.com/medicaid/assisted-living-waivers.*

- For a state-by-state guide to Supplemental Security Income optional state supplements, see *www.payingforseniorcare.com/social-security*.
- In Canada, a private website offers a list of government benefit programs for families of people with dementia. Go to *www.elizz.com/planning/government-assistance-and-funding-for-caregivers-in-canada*.
- In the United Kingdom, you can find out about government benefits for people caring for someone with dementia at *www.nhs.uk/conditions/social-care-and-support-guide/support-and-benefits-for-carers/benefits-for-carers*.
- In Ireland, you can find out about government benefits for people caring for someone with dementia at *www.alzheimer.ie/wp-content/uploads/2020/04/Info-on-HSE-Supports-for-Carers-April-2020.pdf*.

HELP LINES

- The Alzheimer's Association offers a 24-hours-a-day help line for families looking for crisis assistance; decision-making support; treatment options; and answers to financial, legal, and other questions. The help line can also set up a free "care consultation" that can connect you with additional resources that are tailored to your needs. The phone number is (800) 272-3900. There is also a "live chat" option at *www.alz.org/help-support/resources/helpline*. The services are available in a number of languages.
- A similar help line is operated by the Alzheimer's Foundation of America. The phone number is (866) 232-8484, and there is on online chat option at *www.alzfdn.org/afahelpline*. The line is staffed by licensed social workers and is available from 9:00 A.M. to 9:00 P.M. Eastern time 7 days a week.
- The Alzheimer Society of Canada offers a help line at (800) 616-8816.
- In the United Kingdom, the Alzheimer's Society's free support line is 0333 150 3456. Dementia UK also operates a free help line at 0800 888 6678 or *helpline@dementiauk.org*. A Welsh support line is available at 03300 947 400.
- In Ireland, the Alzheimer Society offers a help line at 1800 341 341 or at *helpline@alzheimer.ie*.
- In Australia, the National Dementia help line is available at 1800 100 500 or at *helpline@dementia.org.au*. A webchat is available at *www.dementia.org.au/helpline/webchat*.
- Alzheimers New Zealand offers a help line at 0800 004 001.

HOME CARE SERVICES

* You can find local home care services by going to *www.communityresourcefinder.org* and clicking on "Care at Home," then "Home Care," and entering your zip code.

* For information on Medicaid programs in your state that pay for home care services, go to *www.caregiver.org/connecting-caregivers/services-by-state*, select your state, and click on "Caregiver Compensation."

* In the United Kingdom, you can find home care resources at *www.alzheimers.org.uk/find-support-near-you*. Age UK offers some home care services; see *www.ageuk.org.uk/services/in-your-area/home-help*.

* The Alzheimer Society of Ireland offers home care services at *www.alzheimer.ie/service/home-care-services*.

HOME HEALTH CARE

* A U.S. government website allows you to find home health care services in your area and compare them based on many different criteria. Go to *www.medicare.gov/care-compare*, enter your location, choose "Home health services," and click "Search." Once you see the results, click on the "Compare" button next to all the ones that interest you, then click "Compare" at the upper right.

* You can find local home health care aides and services at *www.communityresourcefinder.org*. Click on "Care at Home," then "Home Health Care," and enter your zip code.

* For information on Medicaid programs in your state that pay for home health care services, go to *www.caregiver.org/connecting-caregivers/services-by-state*, select your state, and click on "Caregiver Compensation."

* In the United Kingdom, you can find home health care resources at *www.alzheimers.org.uk/find-support-near-you*. The Care Quality Commission offers comparative reports on home services providers at *www.cqc.org.uk*.

HOSPICE

* You can find local hospice facilities at *www.communityresourcefinder.org*. Click on "Care at Home," then "Hospice," and enter your zip code.

* You can also find information on hospice programs in your state by going to

www.caregiver.org/connecting-caregivers/services-by-state. Select your state and click on "Resources on Living Arrangements for Care Recipients."

- A U.S. government website allows you to find hospice programs in your area and compare them based on many different criteria. Go to *www.medicare.gov/care-compare*, enter your location, choose "Hospice care," and click "Search." Once you see the results, click on the "Compare" button next to all the ones that interest you, then click "Compare" at the upper right.

- In Ireland, the free "Nurses for Night Care" program can be found at *www.hospicefoundation.ie/our-supports-services/healthcare-hub/nurses-for-night-care.*

- In Australia, a lot of information about hospice services can be found at *www.dementia.org.au/sites/default/files/documents/Dementia-Australia-Numbered-Publication-43.pdf.*

- In New Zealand, you can find local hospice services at *www.hospice.org.nz/what-is-hospice/find-your-local-hospice.*

LEGAL ISSUES

- The National Academy of Elder Law Attorneys is a professional organization of lawyers who specialize in elder law issues. You can find members in your area by going to *www.naela.org/FindALawyer.*

- You can also find local elder law attorneys by going to *www.communityresourcefinder.org* and clicking on "Care at Home," then "Elder Law Attorneys," and entering your zip code.

- If you have trouble affording a lawyer, you can find information on legal-aid programs for people with disabilities (such as dementia) at *www.caregiver.org/connecting-caregivers/services-by-state.* Select your state and click on "Legal Help Advocacy."

- In Canada, you can search for members of the Canadian Bar Association who specialize in elder law at *www.cba.org/For-The-Public/Find-A-Lawyer.* Under "Area of Law," select "Elder Law."

- In the United Kingdom, you can find a lawyer who specializes in elder law at the Solicitors for the Elderly website, *www.sfe.legal/find-a-lawyer.* You can also learn more about dementia-related legal issues at *www.nhs.uk/conditions/dementia/legal-issues.*

- In Ireland, you can search for members of Solicitors for the Elderly Ireland at *www.solicitorsfortheelderly.ie/users/search/new.*

MEMORY CAFÉS

- A "memory café" is a place that allows people with dementia and their care partners to engage in activities together, learn about the disease, and connect with others. To find a memory café in your state, go to *www. memorycafedirectory.com/state-directories*.

- In Canada, go to *www.memorycafedirectory.com/canada*.

- In the United Kingdom, go to *www.memorycafedirectory.com/united-kingdom*.

- In Australia, go to *www.memorycafedirectory.com/australia*.

NURSING HOMES

- A state-by-state guide to finding and comparing nursing homes can be found at *www.seniorliving.org/nursing-homes/state-federal-regulations/#state*.

- Detailed information on Medicare coverage of nursing home care can be found at *www.medicare.gov/Pubs/pdf/10153-Medicare-Skilled-Nursing-Facility-Care.pdf*.

- You can compare nursing homes based on how often they have been cited for regulatory deficiencies at *https://projects.propublica.org/nursing-homes*.

- In Ireland, information on finding and comparing nursing homes can be found at *www.alzheimer.ie/get-support/nursing-home-care-in-ireland*.

SUPPORT GROUPS

- You can find information on state-run and nonprofit family caregiver support programs in your state by going to *www.caregiver.org/connecting-caregivers/services-by-state*, selecting your state, and clicking on "Services Policies for Family Caregivers."

- The Alzheimer's Association offers a large number of support groups for families of people with dementia. Go to *www.alz.org* and click on "Your Chapter" to select your area, then click the link for support groups.

- The Alzheimer's Foundation of America offers telephone-based support groups. You can find information at *www.alzfdn.org/caregiving-resources/2860-2*.

- In Canada, many local branches of the Alzheimer Society offer support groups. You can find your local society's contact information at *www. alzheimer.ca/en/help-support/find-your-society*.

- In the United Kingdom, you can find local support groups at *www. alzheimers.org.uk/find-support-near-you.*

- In Ireland, a list of support groups can be found at *www.alzheimer.ie/service/ support-group.*

- In Australia, an online forum for caregivers can be found at *https://forum. carergateway.gov.au.*

- Many local branches of Alzheimers New Zealand offer support groups. You can find your local branch's contact information at *www.alzheimers.org.nz/ get-support/find-local-help.*

TRANSPORTATION

- You can find information on local transportation options at *www. communityresourcefinder.org.* Click on "Care at Home," then "Transportation," and enter your zip code.

- The U.S. Administration on Aging offers a number of resources for seniors' transportation needs at *www.eldercare.acl.gov/Public/Resources/ LearnMoreAbout/Transportation.aspx.*

- In the United Kingdom, you can find transport resources at *www.alzheimers. org.uk/find-support-near-you.* Also Age UK offers some transport services; see *www.ageuk.org.uk/services/in-your-area/transport.*

- In New Zealand, the "Total Mobility scheme" provides subsidies for transport for people with disabilities. You can find out more at *www.nzta. govt.nz/assets/resources/total-mobility-scheme/docs/total-mobility-around-new-zealand.pdf.*

Notes

Chapter 2. How Can I Know for Sure If My Parent Has Dementia?

PAGES 16–17 • For detailed reviews and analysis of a broad variety of dementia screening tests, see Jennifer S. Lin et al., "Screening for Cognitive Impairment in Older Adults: An Evidence Update for the U.S. Preventive Services Task Force," *Agency for Healthcare Research and Quality (US)* (November 2013), available at *www.ncbi.nlm.nih.gov/books/NBK174641*; Bart Sheehan, "Assessment Scales in Dementia," *Therapeutic Advances in Neurological Disorders* (November 2012): 5(6), 349–358, available at *www.ncbi.nlm.nih.gov/pmc/articles/PMC3487532*.

PAGE 17 • "An even simpler test, called the Mini-Cog, consists of only two tasks: recalling words and drawing a clock face. Despite its simplicity, it has shown fairly good results in diagnosing cognitive impairment." See Andrew Rosenzweig, "How the Mini-Cog Is Used to Test for Alzheimer's and Dementia," available at *www.verywellhealth.com/mini-cog-as-an-alzheimers-screening-test-98622*.

PAGE 17 • For a study of the effectiveness of the GPCOG test, see Eliza Iatraki et al., "Cognitive Screening Tools for Primary Care Settings: Examining the 'Test Your Memory' and 'General Practitioner Assessment of Cognition' Tools in a Rural Aging Population in Greece," *European Journal of General Practice* (2017): 23(1), 171–178, available at *www.ncbi.nlm.nih.gov/pmc/articles/PMC5774277*.

PAGE 18 • "U.S. government figures show that misuse of alcohol and prescription drugs by the elderly is one of the fastest-growing health problems in the country and affects as many as 17 percent of people over age 60." See U.S. Department of Health and Human Services Substance Abuse and Mental Health Services Administration, *Substance Abuse among Older Adults* (October 2012): Chapter 1, available at *www.ncbi.nlm.nih.gov/books/NBK64422*.

PAGE 18 • "One study found that among women over 60, binge drinking increased at an average rate of 3.7 percent per year between 1997 and 2014." See Rosalind A. Breslow et al., "Trends in Alcohol Consumption among Older Americans: National Health Interview Surveys, 1997 to 2014," *Alcoholism: Clinical and Experimental Research* (May 2017): 41(5), 976–986.

PAGE 20 • "One survey asked seniors why they didn't want to be tested . . ." and "Several studies of primary care patients who were offered routine dementia screening found that the refusal rates ranged from 7 to 23 percent." See Malaz Boustani, "Dementia Screening in Primary Care: Not Too Fast!" *Journal of the American Geriatric Society* (July 2013): 61(7), 1205–1207, available at *www.ncbi. nlm.nih.gov/pmc/articles/PMC4167825.*

PAGE 20 • "One survey of residents in affluent retirement communities found that only 49 percent would be willing to be regularly screened for dementia." See Malaz Boustani et al., "Acceptance of Dementia Screening in Continuous Care Retirement Communities: A Mailed Survey," *International Journal of Geriatric Psychiatry* (September 2003): 18(9), 780–786, available at *www.ncbi.nlm.nih.gov/ pubmed/12949845.*

PAGE 21 • "A dementia diagnosis is often more upsetting to family members than it is to the seniors who have dementia." See Robert B. Santulli and Kesstan Blandi, *The Emotional Journey of the Alzheimer's Family* (Lebanon, NH: Dartmouth College Press, 2015), p. 16.

PAGE 21 • "One scientific study found that . . . receiving a dementia diagnosis was highly unlikely to cause seniors to become upset or depressed." See Brian D. Carpenter et al., "Reaction to a Dementia Diagnosis in Individuals with Alzheimer's Disease and Mild Cognitive Impairment," *Journal of the American Geriatric Society* (March 2008): 56(3), 405–412, available at *www.ncbi.nlm.nih.gov/ pubmed/18194228.*

Chapter 3. What Causes Memory Loss?: Alzheimer's Disease and the Many Other Causes

PAGE 23 • "In 2018 a group of scientists conducted autopsies of more than 1,000 people . . ." See Patricia A. Boyle et al., "Person-Specific Contribution of Neuropathologies to Cognitive Loss in Old Age," *Annals of Neurology* (January 2018): 83(1), 74–83, available at *www.ncbi.nlm.nih.gov/pmc/articles/PMC5876116.*

PAGE 24 • "According to the Mayo Clinic . . ." See *www.mayoclinic.org/diseases-conditions/mild-cognitive-impairment/symptoms-causes/syc-20354578.*

PAGES 24–25 • "It's believed that there are currently about 6 million cases of Alzheimer's in the United States, and the number is expected to reach 15 million by 2050." See "2020 Alzheimer's Disease Facts and Figures," *Alzheimer's & Dementia* (2020): *16*, 391–460.

PAGE 28 • "In 2019 a group of scientists proposed that these people actually have a different disease . . ." See Peter T. Nelson et al., "Limbic-Predominant Age-Related TDP-43 Encephalopathy (LATE): Consensus Working Group Report," *Brain* (June 2019): *142*(6), 1503–1527; see also (July 2019): (*142*)7, e37.

Chapter 4. What to Expect: How the Problem Typically Progresses

PAGE 37 • "Families of people with vascular dementia had a much greater caregiving burden in the early stages of the disease compared with families of people with Alzheimer's, but in the later stages the opposite was true." See Peter H. Vetter et al., "Vascular Dementia versus Dementia of Alzheimer's Type: Do They Have Differential Effects on Caregivers' Burden?" *Journal of Gerontology: Social Sciences* (1999): (*54B*)2, S93–S98, available at *https://pdfs.semanticscholar.org/a482/5eecb3962d90c151cdf9712e17b95187e348.pdf.*

Chapter 5. Can Dementia Be Treated to Make It Less Severe?

PAGE 40 • "Some studies have shown that cholinesterase inhibitors are effective for Lewy body dementia." See, for example, Shinji Matsunaga et al., "Cholinesterase Inhibitors for Lewy Body Disorders: A Meta-Analysis," *International Journal of Neuropsychopharmacology* (February 2016): *19*(2), pyv086, available at *www.ncbi.nlm.nih.gov/pmc/articles/PMC4772820.*

PAGE 40 • "The evidence for the use of the drugs with vascular dementia is unclear. Also . . . there may be a risk of adverse drug interactions between cholinesterase inhibitors and common heart medicines." See, for example, Yu-dan Chen et al., "Efficacy of Cholinesterase Inhibitors in Vascular Dementia: An Updated Meta-Analysis," *European Neurology* (2016): *75*(3–4), 132–141, available at *www.ncbi.nlm.nih.gov/pubmed/26918649*; Roger Bullock, "Cholinesterase Inhibitors and Vascular Dementia: Another String to Their Bow?" *CNS Drugs* (2004):*18*(2), 79–92; Babak Tousi, "Should Vascular Dementia Be Treated with Cholinesterase Inhibitors? NO," available at *www.comtecmed.com/cony/2016/Uploads/Editor/Tousi.pdf.*

PAGE 40 • "A recent small study suggested that [Namenda] might help with MCI." See Demet I. Algin et al., "Memantine Improves Semantic Memory in Patients with Amnestic Mild Cognitive Impairment: A Single-Photon Emission Computed Tomography Study," *Journal of International Medical Research* (December 2017): 45(6), 2053–2064, available at *www.ncbi.nlm.nih.gov/pmc/articles/PMC5805216*.

PAGE 40 • "Namenda hasn't been approved for Lewy body or vascular dementia, but a number of studies have shown that it can be effective." See, for example, Oleg S. Levin et al., "Efficacy and Safety of Memantine in Lewy Body Dementia," *Neuroscience and Behavioral Physiology* (July 2009): 39(6), 597–604; Keith A. Wesnes et al., "Memantine Improves Attention and Verbal Episodic Memory in Parkinson's Disease Dementia and Dementia with Lewy Bodies: A Double-Blind, Placebo-Controlled, Multicentre Trial," available at *www.bracketglobal.com/sites/default/files/AAIC-3.pdf*; Andrius Baskys and Anthony C. Hou, "Vascular Dementia: Pharmacological Treatment Approaches and Perspectives," *Clinical Interventions in Aging* (September 2007): 2(3), 327–335, available at *www.ncbi.nlm.nih.gov/pmc/articles/PMC2685259*.

PAGE 41 • "Not much research has been conducted on whether Namenda helps with frontotemporal dementia, but so far there is very little evidence that it does." See Taro Kishi et al., "Memantine for the Treatment of Frontotemporal Dementia: A Meta-Analysis," *Neuropsychiatric Disease and Treatment* (2015): 11, 2883–2885, available at *www.ncbi.nlm.nih.gov/pmc/articles/PMC4648602*.

PAGE 42 • "The decision prompted at least two congressional investigations . . ." See "How an Unproven Alzheimer's Drug Got Approved," *New York Times*, July 19, 2021, available at *www.nytimes.com/2021/07/19/health/alzheimers-drug-aduhelm-fda.html*.

PAGE 42 • "The American Neurological Association issued a press release . . ." See *https://myana.org/publications/news/ana-executive-committee-commentary-fda-approval-aduhelm*.

PAGE 42 • "The president of the Alzheimer's Association stated that he 'welcomes and celebrates . . .'" See *https://dakotahomecare.com/alzheimers-breakthrough-is-just-the-beginning*.

PAGE 42 • "Benzodiazepines . . . can also lead to . . . an increased risk of falling in the elderly." See, for example, Tatjana Bulat et al., "Clinical Practice Algorithms: Medication Management to Reduce Fall Risk in the Elderly—Part 3, Benzodiazepines, Cardiovascular Agents, and Antidepressants," *Journal of the American Academy of Nurse Practitioners* (2008): 20, 56–62. See also generally Paula A. Rochon et al., "The Harms of Benzodiazepines for Patients with

Dementia," *Canadian Medical Association Journal* (April 10, 2017): 189(14), E517–E518.

PAGE 43 • "Again these [sleep] drugs may be helpful, but there are questions about their long-term use." See Philippe Voyer and Lori S. Martin, "Improving Geriatric Mental Health Nursing Care: Making a Case for Going Beyond Psychotropic Medications," *International Journal of Mental Health Nursing* (March 2003): 12(1), 11–21.

PAGE 43 • "Melatonin . . . may also help with sundowning." See Daniel P. Cardinali et al., "Clinical Aspects of Melatonin Intervention in Alzheimer's Disease Progression," *Current Neuropharmacology* (September 2010): 8(3), 218–227. But see also R. Robert Auger et al., "Clinical Practice Guideline for the Treatment of Intrinsic Circadian Rhythm Sleep-Wake Disorders: Advanced Sleep-Wake Phase Disorder (ASWPD), Delayed Sleep-Wake Phase Disorder (DSWPD), Non-24-Hour Sleep-Wake Rhythm Disorder (N24SWD), and Irregular Sleep-Wake Rhythm Disorder (ISWRD). An Update for 2015: An American Academy of Sleep Medicine Clinical Practice Guideline," *Journal of Clinical Sleep Medicine* (October 2015): 11(10), 1199–1236.

PAGE 44 • "Many doctors believe that Seroquel is the least risky antipsychotic for patients with Lewy body dementia." See "Treatment of Lewy Body Dementia," published by the Lewy Body Dementia Association and available at *https://lbda. org/wp-content/uploads/2015/09/treatment.pdf.*

PAGE 44 • "Several studies have suggested that [CBD] can slow the decline of cognitive function in people with dementia and can also calm them down and reduce anxiety, agitation, and behavioral problems." See, for example, Antonio Currais et al., "Amyloid Proteotoxicity Initiates an Inflammatory Response Blocked by Cannabinoids," *Aging and Mechanisms of Disease* (2016): 2(16012), available at *www.nature.com/articles/npjamd201612,* and Shalini Jayant and Bhupesh Sharma, "Selective Modulator of Cannabinoid Receptor Type 2 Reduces Memory Impairment and Infarct Size During Cerebral Hypoperfusion and Vascular Dementia," *Currents in Neurovascular Research* (2016): 13(4), 289–302.

PAGES 44–45 • For a more detailed analysis of psychotherapeutic approaches, see Rakesh K. Tripathi and Sarvada C. Tiwari, "Psychotherapeutic Approaches in the Management of Elderlies with Dementia: An Overview," *Delhi Psychiatry Journal* (April 2009): 12(1), 31–41 and Grazia D'Onofrio et al., "Non-Pharmacological Approaches in the Treatment of Dementia," available at *www.intechopen.com/ books/update-on-dementia/non-pharmacological-approaches-in-the-treatment-of-dementia.*

PAGE 45 • For a study of the effectiveness of problem adaptation therapy, see Dimitris N. Kiosses et al., "Problem Adaptation Therapy (PATH) for Older Adults with Major Depression and Cognitive Impairment: A Randomized Clinical Trial," *JAMA Psychiatry* (January 2015): 72(1), 22–30, available at *www.ncbi.nlm. nih.gov/pmc/articles/PMC4583822.*

PAGE 45 • "There is some evidence that taking melatonin at night can improve cognitive functioning in people with MCI." See Daniel P. Cardinali et al., "Clinical Aspects of Melatonin Intervention in Alzheimer's Disease Progression," *Current Neuropharmacology* (September 2010): 8(3), 218–227.

Chapter 6. Why Caring for Parents with Dementia Is So Much Harder than Caring for Parents with Other Diseases

PAGE 49 • "A study by the Alzheimer's Association . . ." See *Families Care: Alzheimer's Caregiving in the United States 2004*, available at *www.alz.org/national/ documents/report_familiescare.pdf.*

Chapter 9. Your Relationship with Your Other Parent or Stepparent

PAGE 81 • "Statistically women tend to wait longer than men before seeking outside help." See Martin Pinquart and Silvia Sörensen, "Gender Differences in Caregiver Stressors, Social Resources, and Health: An Updated Meta-Analysis," *The Journals of Gerontology: Series B, Psychological Sciences and Social Sciences* (January 2006): 61(1), P33–P45, available at *https://academic.oup.com/ psychsocgerontology/article/61/1/P33/550462.*

Chapter 10. Taking Care of Yourself Is Not an Afterthought

PAGE 90 • "A study at the University of California at Berkeley followed a large group of people with dementia and their families . . ." See Sandy J. Lwi et al., "Poor Caregiver Mental Health Predicts Mortality of Patients with Neurodegenerative Disease," *Proceedings of the National Academy of Sciences of the United States of America* (July 2017): 114(28), available at *www.ncbi.nlm.nih. gov/pmc/articles/PMC5514722.* See also *www.healthline.com/health-news/caregiver- mental-stress-shortens-dementia-patients-lives#1.*

Chapter 14. When Is It Okay to Lie to Your Parent?

PAGE 125 • "One scientific study found that receiving a formal dementia diagnosis was very unlikely to cause seniors to become depressed or upset." See Brian D. Carpenter et al., "Reaction to a Dementia Diagnosis in Individuals with Alzheimer's Disease and Mild Cognitive Impairment," *Journal of the American Geriatric Society* (March 2008): 56(3), 405–412, available at *www.ncbi.nlm.nih.gov/pubmed/18194228.*

Chapter 16. Getting Help When Your Parent Lives at Home or with You

PAGE 139 • "There are more than 5,600 adult day centers in the United States, and almost 80 percent of them operate on a nonprofit basis. The average age of participants is 72, and about two-thirds are women. One study found that slightly more than half of all participants have some form of cognitive impairment." See the 2010 MetLife National Study of Adult Day Centers, summarized at *www.nadsa.org/consumers/overview-and-facts.* See also *www.seniorliving.org/adult-day-care.*

Chapter 19. How to Reduce Problem Behaviors

PAGE 159 • For a discussion of sleep problems and dementia, see Cynthia L. Deschenes and Susan M. McCurry, "Current Treatments for Sleep Disturbances in Individuals With Dementia," *Current Psychiatry Reports* (February 2009): 11(1), 20–26, available at *www.ncbi.nlm.nih.gov/pmc/articles/PMC2649672.*

Chapter 24. How Am I Going to Pay for All This?

PAGE 198 • "You might be able to avoid the 3-day rule . . ." For more details, see *www.cms.gov/medicare/medicare-fee-for-service-payment/sharedsavingsprogram/downloads/snf-waiver-guidance.pdf.*

PAGE 199 • For a state-by-state guide to SSI optional state supplements, see *www.payingforseniorcare.com/social-security.*

PAGE 201 • For a state-by-state guide to Medicaid waiver programs for dementia care in assisted-living facilities, see *www.dementiacarecentral.com/medicaid/assisted-living-waivers.*

Chapter 26. Dealing with the End of Life

PAGE 213 • "Alzheimer's disease is the sixth most common cause of death in the United States, according to the Centers for Disease Control and Prevention." See *www.cdc.gov/nchs/fastats/leading-causes-of-death.htm.*

PAGE 213 • "Between 2000 and 2018, the number of people dying from Alzheimer's disease increased by 146 percent . . ." *Alzheimer's Disease 2020 Facts and Figures,* annual report released by the Alzheimer's Association; see *www.alz. org/alzheimers-dementia/facts-figures.*

PAGE 213 • "One study in the journal *Alzheimer's & Dementia* . . ." See "2014 Alzheimer's Disease Facts and Figures," *Alzheimer's & Dementia* (March 2014): 10 (2), available at *www.sciencedirect.com/science/article/pii/S1552526014000624.*

PAGE 213 • "A separate study in the journal *Neurology* . . ." See *Neurology* (March 5, 2014), summarized at *www.aan.com/PressRoom/Home/PressRelease/1253.* See also generally National Institute on Aging, "Number of Alzheimer's Deaths Found To Be Underreported," (May 22, 2014), available at *www.nia.nih.gov/news/ number-alzheimers-deaths-found-be-underreported.*

PAGE 215 • "More than 55 percent of hospice care was provided in a home environment." See National Hospice and Palliative Care Organization Facts and Figures, 2017 edition (revised April 2018), p. 6; available at *https://39k5cm1a9u1968hg74aj3x51-wpengine.netdna-ssl.com/wp-content/ uploads/2019/04/2017_Facts_Figures-2.pdf.*

PAGE 215 • "The humorist Art Buchwald . . ." See Louis Sahagun, "Humorist Got Last Laugh on Death," *Los Angeles Times,* January 19, 2007.

PAGE 215 • "One scientific study showed that patients who received hospice care lived longer than similar patients who didn't." Stephen R. Connor et al., "Comparing Hospice and Nonhospice Patient Survival Among Patients Who Die within a Three-Year Window," *Journal of Pain and Symptom Management* (2007): 33(3), 238–246.

PAGES 215–216 • "One survey of hospice providers found that this uncertainty is the leading reason why hospice services are underutilized for dementia patients." See Karen Appold, "Hospice for Dementia Patients," *Today's Geriatric Medicine,* available at *www.todaysgeriatricmedicine.com/news/ex_042512.shtml.*

Index

About the Authors

Thomas F. Harrison is a professional writer and the former editor of a leading national periodical for attorneys. He has extensive personal experience caring for family members with dementia. Based in Massachusetts, he is the coauthor of *The Complete Family Guide to Addiction.*

Brent P. Forester, MD, is Chief of Geriatric Psychiatry at McLean Hospital in Belmont, Massachusetts, and Associate Professor of Psychiatry at Harvard Medical School. He is also Senior Medical Director for Population Health Management at Mass General Brigham, where he leads a systemwide dementia-care program. Dr. Forester's award-winning research focuses on developing and testing effective treatments for dementia and mood disorders in older adults.